Programmed Mathematics for Nurses

Programmed Mathematics for Nurses

George I. Sackheim

Science Instructor, St. Francis Hospital School of Nursing, Evanston, Illinois. Associate Professor Emeritus of Chemistry, University of Illinois at Chicago. Formerly Lecturer, School of Health Sciences, Michael Reese Hospital and Medical Center, Chicago. Coordinator of Biological and Physical Sciences, School of Nursing, Michael Reese Hospital and Medical Center, Chicago. Science Instructor, School of Nursing, Presbyterian–St. Luke's Hospital, Chicago.

Lewis Robins

President, Creative Learning, Inc., Westport, Conn. Consulting Systems Analyst, Radiology Department, Orthopaedic Institute, New York City.

Fifth Edition

MACMILLAN PUBLISHING CO., INC.
New York

Collier Macmillan Canada, Inc.
Toronto

Collier Macmillan Publishers
London

Macmillan Publishing Co., Inc.
866 Third Avenue, New York, New York 10022

Collier Macmillan Canada, Inc.

Collier Macmillan Publishers · London

Library of Congress Cataloging in Publication Data

Sackheim, George I.
　　Programmed mathematics for nurses.

　　1. Nursing—Mathematics—Programmed　instruction. 2. Pharmaceutical arithmetic—Programmed instruction. I. Robins, Lewis. II. Title.
RT68.S23 1983　　　615′.14　　　82–20355
ISBN 0–02–405170–5

Printing:　2 3 4 5 6 7 8 9 0　　Year: 3 4 5 6 7 8 9 0 1 2

Preface

A New Way to Learn the Mathematics of Nursing

Here is an enjoyable way to learn the mathematics of nursing. In numerous tests, we have determined that a relaxed student, using this pleasant new system, can learn to solve the many types of problems that may be encountered in the giving of medications and in the preparation of solutions. Its purpose is to show that the mathematics of nursing is not something to be afraid of, but rather an old friend that we are now using for problems in nursing.

The secret lies in a group of new psychological principles that make up the *reinforced learning system*. These new principles were discovered in psychological experiments conducted in the laboratories of Columbia and Harvard universities, and we acknowledge with warm thanks the debt we owe to the team of professors led by Fred S. Keller and William N. Schoenfeld of the Department of Psychology, Columbia University, and to B. F. Skinner of Harvard University, who over a period of years developed the underlying principles that we applied in creating this new training method.

Unlike an ordinary text that must be studied and memorized, this *reinforced learning* course asks the student to solve a logical series of problems. After responding to each problem, the student reads the answer to see immediately if she is correct.

Each problem is designed to stimulate the student to *think out* the correct answer on the basis of information she has already learned. Sometimes the student's response will be incorrect. However, because she reads the correct answer immediately after making a mistake, she will learn quickly and easily.

This book presents a wealth of detailed information but, because each concept is broken down into a series of interesting questions and problems, the student will be able to master the most difficult subjects without tedious rote learning.

About the Fifth Edition

Programmed Mathematics for Nurses includes 18 chapters dealing with various aspects of the subjects of units and measurements, and miscellaneous medications and procedures. Three appendixes are also included. At three points in the text you will be given an opportunity to review by means of practice tests.

Included in the fifth edition is a section on IV deficits, and also problems involving microgram dosages. Since more and more hospitals are using computers for all types of purposes, the chapter on computers has been completely revised and updated, with a special emphasis on *drug interactions*. In addition, computer printouts for medication orders have been used throughout the book in order to give the student direct examples of the types of medication problems that will be encountered in hospital situations.

The apothecaries' system, although no longer taught in medical and nursing schools, is still used in some hospitals. Therefore, the section on the apothecaries' system has been taken out of the main text and placed in an appendix. Practice tests in the apothecaries' system also appear there.

Don't Worry if You Make Mistakes

Adults learn from their mistakes. Our experience with the reinforced learning system shows that the number of errors a student makes does not necessarily indicate her ability. As long as the student is immediately aware that she has made a mistake, she will quickly learn to make the correct response. Therefore, don't worry if you make errors.

We believe that your reinforced learning course in the mathematics of nursing offers the best and easiest way to learn the subject, and we wish you success in taking the course.

Acknowledgments

The authors wish to express their appreciation to the following persons for their invaluable assistance in the preparation of the fifth edition:

Dr. Bruce Cohen, Northwestern University Medical Center, Chicago, Ill.

Miss Susan Hogan, Instructor, School of Nursing, South Chicago Community Hospital, Chicago, Ill.

Miss Lois M. Horton, Instructor, School of Nursing, Lutheran General Hospital, Park Ridge, Ill.

Mr. Ronald Kaminski, Director of Pharmacology, Greenwich Hospital, Greenwich, Conn.

Mr. Aaron Kaplan, Chief Pharmacist, Mile Square Health Center, Chicago, Ill.

Miss Virginia Lapie, Educational Director, School of Nursing, South Chicago Community Hospital, Chicago, Ill.

Dr. E. Laska, Director, Information Sciences Division, Rockland Research Institute, Orangeburg, N.Y.

Mr. C. C. Lev, Chief Pharmacist, Michael Reese Hospital and Medical Center, Chicago, Ill.

Miss Mary Lyons, Instructor, School of Nursing, St. Francis Hospital, Evanston, Ill.

Miss Clare O'Boyle, Associate Director, School of Nursing, St. Francis Hospital, Evanston, Ill.

Miss Anne Lynn Porter, Assistant Chairman for Education and Research, Department of Nursing, Evanston Hospital, Evanston, Ill.

Miss Estelle Rogers, Vice President, Nursing Education, School of Nursing, St. Francis Hospital, Evanston, Ill.

Dr. Carole Siegel, Rockland Research Institute, Orangeburg, N.Y.

Mr. Jeff Slater, Senior Systems Analyst, Astradyne Corp., Garden City, N.Y.

Miss Mary Jane Sparrow, Instructor, School of Nursing, St. Francis Hospital, Evanston, Ill.

Contents

UNIT One

Units and Measurements

UNIT Two

**Miscellaneous Medications
and Procedures**

Appendixes

Instructions

Note: These Instructions Must Be Followed Exactly

You will need pencil and paper as well as the RED ACETATE CARD (which is stored in the envelope pasted inside the front cover).

1. Look at page 1 and notice the red rectangular areas. These areas contain answers to the problems.

2. Starting at the top of the page, read the first paragraph.

3. Write $3 \div 5$ as a fraction.

4. Cover the red rectangular area to the right with your RED ACETATE CARD. Notice that the correct answer appears. If you have made a mistake, draw a circle around your incorrect answer.

5. Read the next question.

6. Write your answer.

7. Place your RED ACETATE CARD over the red rectangular area to see if you are correct. If you have made a mistake, draw a circle around your answer. These are the simple reinforced learning procedures. Notice that as soon as you write an answer, you have the *immediate satisfaction* of knowing whether you are correct. If you find that you have made a mistake, you will quickly learn not to repeat it.

8. Now, following the same procedures, complete each of the problems in Section 1.

What to Do After Completing Section 1

1. Count your errors.

2. Passing score is no more than *3* errors.

3. If you fail to achieve a passing score, repeat the section.

Fractions

Units and Measurements

Section 1   Multiplying a Fraction by a Whole Number

A fraction represents one number divided by another number. For instance, the fraction $\frac{2}{3}$ represents *2 divided by 3*.

Express each of the following as fractions:

1. $3 \div 5$ $\frac{3}{5}$

2. $5 \div 7$ $\frac{5}{7}$

3. $18 \div 61$ $\frac{18}{61}$

4. $2 \div 9$ $\frac{2}{9}$

Look at the following fraction carefully:

$$\frac{3}{4}$$

The number above the line is called the numerator; the number below the line is called the denominator.

5. What is the numerator of $\frac{3}{4}$?

Remember that the number above the line is called the numerator.

6. What is the numerator of $\frac{9}{13}$?

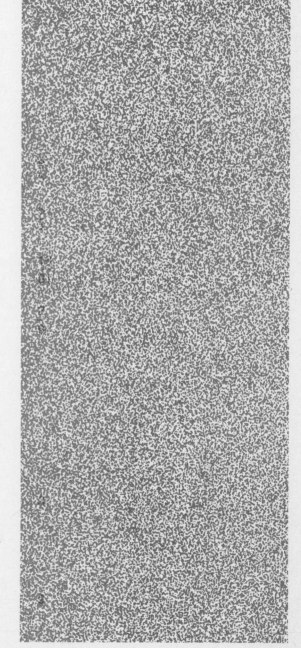

7. What is the denominator of $\frac{3}{4}$?

Remember that the denominator is the number below the line.

8. What is the numerator of $\frac{16}{41}$?

9. What is the numerator of $\frac{27}{95}$?

10. What is the denominator of $\frac{43}{157}$?

Now let us consider how to multiply a fraction by a whole number.

Notice the two steps for multiplying $\frac{2}{3} \times 6$.

Step 1:   Multiply the numerator by the whole number.

$$\frac{2}{3} \times 6 = \frac{12}{3}$$

Step 2:   Divide the result by the denominator.

$$\frac{12}{3} = 4$$

That's all there is to it.

To multiply a fraction by a whole number, multiply the numerator by the whole number and divide the new fraction by the denominator.

Multiply each of the following examples.

11. $\frac{1}{3} \times 9 = \frac{9}{3} = 3$

12. $\frac{1}{2} \times 8 = \frac{8}{2} = 4$

13. $\frac{2}{3} \times 18 = \frac{36}{3} = 12$

14. $\frac{2}{9} \times 27 = \frac{34}{9} = 6$

15. $\frac{4}{5} \times 10 = \frac{40}{5} = 8$

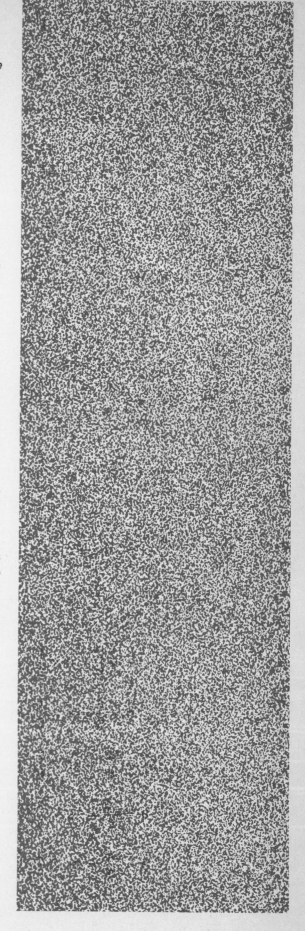

16. $\dfrac{1}{6} \times 24 = \dfrac{24}{6} = 4$

17. $\dfrac{3}{8} \times 16 = \dfrac{6}{1} = 6$

18. $\dfrac{2}{7} \times 14 = 4$

Passing score is no more than *2* errors. If you failed to achieve a passing score, repeat the section.

Section 2   Simplifying Improper Fractions

Look at the following fraction:

$$\frac{24}{5}$$

Notice that the numerator is larger than the denominator. Whenever the numerator is larger than the denominator, the fraction is known as an *improper fraction*.

Look at the following number.

$$2\frac{1}{2}$$

Whenever a number consists of a whole number and a fraction, it is known as a *mixed number*.

Let us consider the procedures for simplifying an improper fraction.

Look at the following fraction:

$$\frac{25}{4}$$

Bear in mind that $\dfrac{25}{4}$ represents 25 divided by 4.

1. Can 25 be divided evenly by 4?   *no*

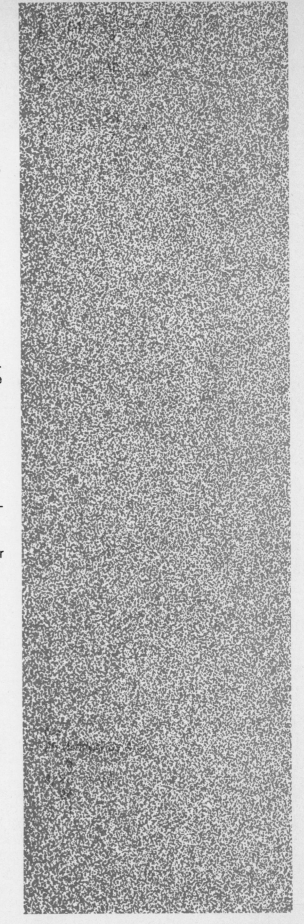

Here is how to simplify an improper fraction:

Divide the numerator by the denominator. If the numerator cannot be divided evenly by the denominator, express the result as a mixed number.

Let us try several problems.

Express each of the following improper fractions as mixed numbers.

2. $\dfrac{31}{5} = 6\frac{1}{5}$

3. $\dfrac{25}{8} = 3\frac{1}{8}$

4. $\dfrac{53}{9} = 5\frac{8}{9}$

5. $\dfrac{49}{8} = 6\frac{1}{8}$

6. $\dfrac{79}{11} = 7\frac{2}{11}$

7. $\dfrac{81}{8} = 10\frac{1}{8}$

8. $\dfrac{53}{7} = 7\frac{4}{7}$

9. $\dfrac{15}{8} = 1\frac{7}{8}$

10. $\dfrac{26}{5} = 5\frac{1}{5}$

Read the following carefully:

$$\frac{3}{8} \times 5 = \frac{15}{8} = 1\frac{7}{8}$$

Whenever you are multiplying fractions, if the result is an improper fraction, divide the numerator by the denominator. If the numerator of the result cannot be evenly divided by the denominator, express the result as a mixed number.

Let us try several problems.

Multiply the following numbers.

11. $\dfrac{2}{3} \times 10 = \dfrac{20}{3} = 6\,2/3$

12. $\dfrac{5}{7} \times 9 = \dfrac{45}{7} = 6\,3/7$

13. $\dfrac{3}{8} \times 5 = \dfrac{15}{8} = 1\,7/8$

14. $\dfrac{5}{12} \times 7 = \dfrac{35}{12} = 2\,11/12$

15. $\dfrac{6}{11} \times 5 = \dfrac{30}{11} = 2\,8/11$

16. $\dfrac{3}{8} \times 9 = \dfrac{27}{8} = 3\,3/8$

Passing score is no more than *2* errors.

Section 3 Multiplying Two Fractions

To multiply two fractions, multiply their numerators and also multiply their denominators.

For example:

$$\frac{1}{2} \times \frac{3}{4} = \frac{1 \times 3}{2 \times 4} = \frac{3}{8}$$

Let us try a few problems.

Multiply each of the following fractions.

1. $\dfrac{5}{6} \times \dfrac{1}{3} = \dfrac{5}{18}$

2. $\dfrac{7}{4} \times \dfrac{1}{8} = \dfrac{7}{32}$

3. $\dfrac{8}{9} \times \dfrac{1}{5} = \dfrac{8}{45}$

4. $\dfrac{3}{5} \times \dfrac{1}{7} = \dfrac{3}{35}$

5. $\dfrac{1}{4} \times \dfrac{3}{5} = \dfrac{3}{20}$

6. $\frac{5}{7} \times \frac{6}{11} = \frac{30}{77}$

7. $\frac{1}{3} \times \frac{11}{9} = \frac{11}{27}$

8. $\frac{7}{13} \times \frac{2}{3} = \frac{14}{39}$

Passing score is no more than *1* error.

Section 4   Simplifying Fractions

Read the following example carefully.

$$\frac{7}{8} \times \frac{5}{4} = \frac{35}{32} = 1\frac{3}{32}$$

Whenever the result of multiplying two fractions is an improper fraction, the result is simplified by changing it to a mixed number.

1. Simplify $\frac{35}{32}$ by changing it to a mixed number.

2. Multiply and simplify $\frac{11}{4} \times \frac{3}{7}$.

Multiply each of the following fractions and express the answers as mixed numbers.

3. $\frac{27}{4} \times \frac{1}{5} = \frac{27}{20} = 1\frac{7}{20}$

4. $\frac{17}{5} \times \frac{3}{4} = \frac{51}{20} = 2\frac{11}{20}$

5. $\frac{7}{13} \times \frac{5}{2} = \frac{35}{26} = 1\frac{9}{26}$

6. $\frac{6}{7} \times \frac{11}{5} = \frac{66}{35} = 1\frac{31}{35}$

7. $\frac{21}{2} \times \frac{1}{4} = \frac{21}{8} = 2\frac{5}{8}$

8. $\frac{19}{3} \times \frac{1}{2} = \frac{19}{6} = 3\frac{1}{6}$

9. $\frac{9}{2} \times \frac{5}{4} = \frac{45}{8} = 5\frac{5}{8}$

10. $\dfrac{7}{8} \times \dfrac{9}{1} = \dfrac{63}{8} = 7\dfrac{7}{8}$

Passing score is no more than *1* error.

Section 5   Simplifying Fractions (cont.)

Look at the diagrams below.

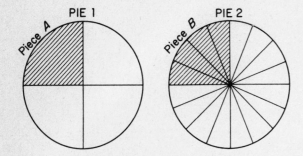

1.   Into how many pieces has Pie 1 been divided?

2.   How would you describe the size of Piece A?

3.   Into how many pieces has Pie 2 been divided?

4.   How would you describe the size of Piece B?

Look again at the diagrams.

Notice that A and B are exactly the same size. However, describing the size of the piece as $\dfrac{1}{4}$ is simpler than describing it as $\dfrac{4}{16}$.

Read the following carefully.

$$\frac{3}{8} \times \frac{1}{3} = \frac{3}{24}$$

However, $\dfrac{3}{24} = \dfrac{1}{8}$.

The result of multiplying two fractions is usually expressed in the simplest terms.

Let us find out how to reduce a proper fraction to its simplest terms.

Consider the following fraction:

$$\frac{2}{4}$$

5. What is the largest number by which the numerator and the denominator can both be divided *evenly*?

Notice what happens when both the numerator and denominator are divided by 2.

$$\frac{2 \div 2}{4 \div 2} = \frac{1}{2}$$

Consider the following fraction:

$$\frac{4}{8}$$

6. What is the largest number by which the numerator and denominator can both be divided *evenly*?

Notice what happens when both the numerator and denominator are divided by 4.

$$\frac{4 \div 4}{8 \div 4} = \frac{1}{2}$$

To reduce any fraction, try to find the largest number by which both the numerator and denominator can be divided evenly. Dividing the numerator and denominator by the same number reduces the fraction.

Let us try a few problems. Consider the following fraction:

$$\frac{3}{9}$$

7. What is the largest number by which both the numerator and denominator can be evenly divided?

Consider the following fraction:

$$\frac{5}{15}$$

8. What is the largest number by which both the numerator and denominator can be evenly divided?

9. Reduce the fraction to its simplest terms by dividing both the numerator and denominator by 5.

Consider the following fraction:

$$\frac{12}{16}$$

10. What is the largest number by which both the numerator and denominator can be evenly divided?

11. Reduce the fraction to its simplest terms by dividing both the numerator and denominator by 4.

12. Reduce $\frac{6}{9}$ to its simplest terms.

13. Reduce $\frac{6}{8}$ to its simplest terms.

Reduce each of the following fractions to its simplest terms.

14. $\frac{7}{49} = \frac{1}{7}$

15. $\frac{4}{12} = \frac{1}{3}$

16. $\frac{8}{10} = \frac{4}{5}$

17. $\frac{10}{25} = \frac{2}{5}$

18. $\frac{3}{9} = \frac{1}{3}$

19. $\dfrac{24}{42} = \dfrac{4}{7}$

20. $\dfrac{16}{20} = \dfrac{4}{5}$

21. $\dfrac{14}{42} = \dfrac{1}{3}$

22. $\dfrac{80}{100} = \dfrac{4}{5}$

Passing score is no more than *2* errors.

Section 6 Simplifying Fractions (cont.)

Look at the following fraction:

$$\frac{28}{36}$$

Notice that the numbers in the numerator and denominator are rather large. Because the numbers are large, you may find it difficult to determine the *largest* number by which both the numerator and denominator can be divided evenly.

Here's all you do.

Notice that the numerator and denominator are even numbers. Therefore, the fraction can be reduced by dividing both numerator and denominator by 2. For example:

$$\frac{28}{36} = \frac{14}{18}$$

Notice that the numerator and denominator are still even numbers. Therefore, the fraction can be further simplified by dividing again by 2.

$$\frac{14}{18} = \frac{7}{9}$$

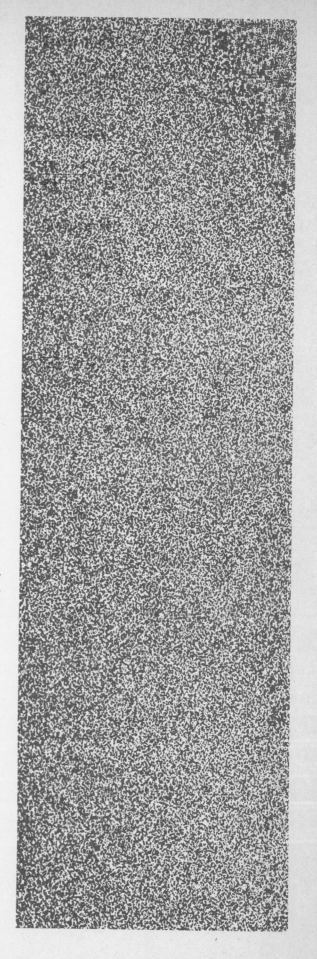

In this way, the fraction $\frac{28}{36}$ has been reduced to its lowest terms.

Let's consider another example.

Assume that you want to reduce the following fraction to its lowest terms.

$$\frac{36}{44}$$

Because the numbers are large, you may find it difficult to determine the *largest* number by which both the numerator and denominator can be divided evenly.

1. Therefore, first reduce the fraction by dividing both the numerator and denominator by 2. $\frac{36}{44} = \frac{18}{22} = \frac{9}{11}$

2. Reduce the fraction to its simplest terms.

Let's try another example.

Look at the following fraction.

$$\frac{136}{176} \div \frac{2}{2} =$$

3. First reduce the fraction by dividing by 2. $\frac{68}{88} \div \frac{2}{2} =$

4. Since the fraction is still large, reduce the fraction by dividing by 2. $\frac{34}{44} \div \frac{2}{2} =$

5. Once again, divide by 2. $\frac{17}{22}$

Remember that if both the numerator and denominator are even numbers, you can always simplify the fraction by dividing both the numerator and denominator by 2.

Reduce each of the following fractions to its simplest terms.

6. $\frac{56}{96} = \frac{28}{48} = \frac{14}{24} = \frac{7}{12}$

7. $\frac{24}{68} = \frac{12}{34} = \frac{6}{17}$

8. $\frac{20}{36} = \frac{10}{18} = \frac{5}{9}$

9. $\dfrac{48}{64} = \dfrac{24}{32} = \dfrac{6}{8} = \dfrac{3}{4}$

10. $\dfrac{64}{128} = \dfrac{1}{2}$

11. $\dfrac{68}{112} = \dfrac{34}{56} = \dfrac{17}{28}$

12. $\dfrac{16}{24} = \dfrac{8}{12} = \dfrac{2}{3}$

13. $\dfrac{100}{252} = \dfrac{50}{126} = \dfrac{25}{63}$

14. $\dfrac{36}{64} = \dfrac{18}{32} = \dfrac{9}{16}$

15. $\dfrac{92}{132} = \dfrac{46}{66} = \dfrac{23}{33}$

16. $\dfrac{148}{216} = \dfrac{74}{108} = \dfrac{37}{54}$

17. $\dfrac{200}{228} = \dfrac{100}{114} = \dfrac{50}{57}$

Passing score is no more than *2* errors.

Section 7 Simplifying Fractions (cont.)

Look at the following fraction:

$$\frac{126}{153}$$

Because the numbers are large, you may find it difficult to determine the largest number by which both the numerator and denominator can be divided evenly.

In that case, here's all you do.

Notice that the denominator is an odd number. Whenever the numerator or the denominator is an odd number, the fraction cannot be reduced by dividing by 2. However, you may be able to reduce the fraction by dividing by 3. For example:

$$\frac{126 \div 3}{153 \div 3} = \frac{42}{51}$$

Notice that the denominator is still an odd number.

Possibly the fraction can be further reduced by dividing again by 3.

$$\frac{42 \div 3}{51 \div 3} = \frac{14}{17}$$

In this way, the fraction $\frac{126}{153}$ is reduced to its lowest terms.

Let us consider another example. Assume you want to reduce the following fraction to its lowest terms.

$$\frac{99}{198}$$

Because the numbers are large, you may find it difficult to determine the *largest* number by which both the numerator and denominator can be divided evenly.

1. Therefore, first try to reduce the fraction by dividing both the numerator and denominator by 3.

2. Reduce the fraction to its simplest terms.

Let us try more examples. Reduce each of the following fractions to their simplest terms.

3. $\frac{93}{186} = \frac{31}{62}$

4. $\frac{45}{90} = \frac{15}{30} = \frac{1}{2}$

5. $\frac{81}{108} = \frac{27}{36} = \frac{9}{12} = \frac{3}{4}$

6. $\frac{54}{189} = \frac{18}{63} = \frac{6}{21} = \frac{2}{7}$

7. $\frac{189}{216} = \frac{63}{72} = \frac{7}{8}$

8. $\frac{27}{243} = \frac{9}{81} = \frac{1}{9}$

9. $\frac{81}{135} = \frac{27}{45} = \frac{9}{15} = \frac{3}{5}$

10. $\frac{90}{117} = \frac{30}{39} = \frac{10}{13}$

11. $\frac{27}{162} = \frac{3}{18} = \frac{1}{6}$

12. $\dfrac{135}{189} = \dfrac{45}{63} = \dfrac{5}{7}$

13. $\dfrac{54}{243} = \dfrac{6}{27} = \dfrac{2}{9}$

14. $\dfrac{108}{135} = \dfrac{136}{45} = \dfrac{4}{5}$

15. $\dfrac{108}{189} = \dfrac{36}{63} = \dfrac{4}{7}$

16. $\dfrac{189}{270} = \dfrac{63}{90} = \dfrac{7}{10}$

17. $\dfrac{27}{189} = \dfrac{9}{63} = \dfrac{3}{21} = \dfrac{1}{7}$

18. $\dfrac{162}{243} = \dfrac{18}{27} = \dfrac{2}{3}$

19. $\dfrac{135}{270} = \dfrac{45}{90} = \dfrac{5}{10} = \frac{1}{2}$

Passing score is no more than *3* errors.

Section 8   Multiplying Two Fractions

Multiply the following fractions and reduce the answers to the simplest terms.

1. $\dfrac{2}{3} \times \dfrac{4}{6} = \dfrac{4}{9}$

2. $\dfrac{4}{9} \times \dfrac{3}{2} = \dfrac{2}{3}$

3. $\dfrac{1}{11} \times \dfrac{2}{8} = \dfrac{1}{44}$

4. $\dfrac{3}{10} \times \dfrac{1}{12} = \dfrac{1}{40}$

5. $\dfrac{15}{30} \times \dfrac{2}{5} = \dfrac{1}{5}$

6. $\dfrac{3}{4} \times \dfrac{1}{18} = \dfrac{1}{24}$

7. $\dfrac{8}{7} \times \dfrac{3}{4} = \dfrac{6}{7}$

8. $\dfrac{7}{9} \times \dfrac{5}{10} = \dfrac{7}{18}$

9. $\dfrac{12}{25} \times \dfrac{5}{3} = \dfrac{4}{5}$

10. $\dfrac{2}{7} \times \dfrac{5}{12} = \dfrac{5}{42}$

11. $\dfrac{4}{8} \times \dfrac{5}{10} = \dfrac{1}{4}$

12. $\dfrac{3}{10} \times \dfrac{5}{8} = \dfrac{3}{16}$

13. $\dfrac{2}{15} \times \dfrac{1}{4} = \dfrac{1}{30}$

14. $\dfrac{27}{72} \times \dfrac{4}{3} = \dfrac{1}{2}$

Passing score is no more than *3* errors.

Section 9   How to Change a Mixed Number to a Fraction

Consider the following problem:

$$\frac{3}{4} \times 3\frac{15}{16}$$

Notice that the problem is to multiply a fraction by a mixed number. Whenever you want to multiply a fraction by a mixed number, the first step is to change the mixed number to an improper fraction.

Here is all you do.

Mixed Number	Step 1
$3\frac{15}{16}$	$3 \times 16 = 48$

Step 2	Step 3 Improper Fraction
$48 + 15 = 63$	$\dfrac{63}{16}$

Look at the above chart.

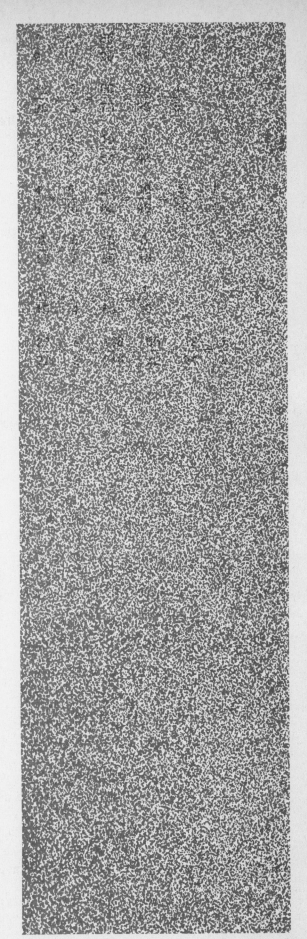

1. What is the denominator of the fraction in the mixed number?

Look at Step 1.

Notice that the whole number is multiplied by the denominator. The product is 48.

2. What is the numerator of the mixed number?

Look at Step 2.

Notice that the numerator is added to the product. The sum is 63.

Look at Step 3.

Notice that the sum is placed over the denominator.

That is all there is to changing a mixed number to an improper fraction.

Now let us try another example.

Be sure you follow the step-by-step procedures.

Consider the following fraction:

$$5\frac{13}{16}$$

3. Step 1. Multiply the whole number by the denominator.

4. Step 2. Add the numerator to the product.

5. Step 3. Place the sum over the denominator.

That is all there is to it.

Let's try another example.

Consider the following fraction:

$$12\frac{5}{7}$$

6. Step 1. Multiply the whole number by the denominator.

7. Step 2. Add the numerator to the product.

8. Step 3. Place the sum over the denominator.

Change each of the following mixed numbers to improper fractions.

9. $11\frac{2}{3} = \frac{35}{3}$

10. $5\frac{3}{4} = \frac{23}{4}$

11. $9\frac{3}{5} = \frac{48}{5}$

12. $14\frac{1}{2} = \frac{29}{2}$

13. $3\frac{8}{9} = \frac{35}{9}$

14. $4\frac{2}{3} = \frac{14}{3}$

15. $7\frac{1}{4} = \frac{29}{4}$

16. $9\frac{1}{2} = \frac{19}{2}$

17. $8\frac{3}{4} = \frac{35}{4}$

18. $6\frac{7}{8} = \frac{55}{8}$

19. $1\frac{3}{7} = \frac{10}{7}$

20. $9\frac{1}{3} = \frac{28}{3}$

Passing score is no more than *3* errors.

Section 10   How to Multiply a Mixed Number by a Fraction

Consider the following problem:

$$4\frac{16}{29} \times \frac{2}{3}$$

Notice that the problem is to multiply a mixed number by a fraction. Here is all you do.

Problem	**Step 1 Change Mixed Number to Improper Fraction**
$4\frac{16}{29} \times \frac{2}{3}$	$4\frac{16}{29} = \frac{132}{29}$

Step 2 Multiply	**Step 3 Change Result to Mixed Number**
$\frac{132}{29} \times \frac{2}{3} = \frac{264}{87}$	$\frac{264}{87} = \frac{88}{29} = 3\frac{1}{29}$

Look at the above chart.

1. What is the first step?

2. What is the second step?

3. What is the third step?

18 UNITS AND MEASUREMENTS

Let us try several examples. Be sure to follow the step-by-step procedures.

Consider the following problem:

$$10\frac{2}{3} \times \frac{9}{10}$$

4. Step 1. Change the mixed number to an improper fraction.

5. Step 2. Multiply the fractions.

6. Step 3. Change the result to a mixed number.

Let us try another example.

Consider the following problem:

$$14\frac{7}{8} \times \frac{1}{2}$$

7. Step 1. Change the mixed number to an improper fraction.

8. Step 2. Multiply the fractions.

9. Step 3. Change the result to a mixed number.

Solve each of the following problems.

10. $10\frac{1}{2} \times \frac{1}{2}$

$$\frac{21}{2} \times \frac{1}{2} = \frac{21}{4}$$

$$4\overline{)21} = 5\frac{1}{4}$$
$$\frac{20}{1}$$

11. $2\frac{1}{6} \times \frac{2}{3}$

$$\frac{13}{6} \times \frac{2}{3} = \frac{13}{9}$$

$$9\overline{)13} = 1\frac{4}{9}$$

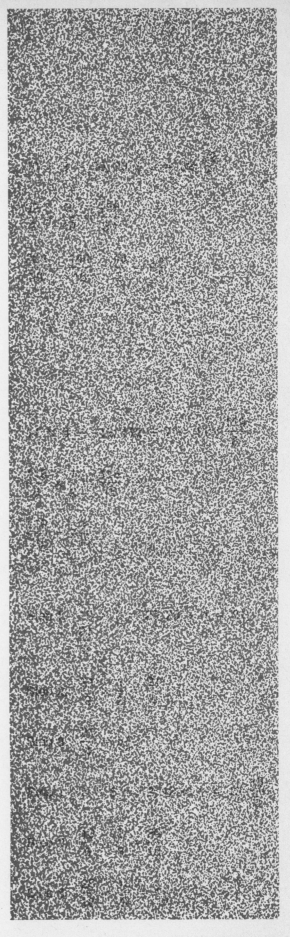

12. $8\frac{1}{4} \times \frac{1}{2}$

$\frac{33}{4} \times \frac{1}{2} = \frac{33}{8}$

$8\overline{)33} \quad = 4\frac{1}{8}$
$\quad\underline{32}$
$\quad\ 1$

13. $5\frac{6}{7} \times \frac{3}{5}$

$\frac{41}{7} \times \frac{3}{5} = \frac{123}{35}$

$35\overline{)123} = 3\frac{18}{35}$
$\quad\underline{105}$
$\quad\ 18$

14. $7\frac{3}{8} \times \frac{3}{4}$ $\frac{59}{8} \times \frac{3}{4} = \frac{177}{32}$ $32\overline{)177} = 5\frac{17}{32}$
$\qquad\qquad\qquad\qquad\qquad\quad \underline{160}$
$\qquad\qquad\qquad\qquad\qquad\quad\ \ 17$

15. $4\frac{3}{8} \times \frac{1}{5}$ $\frac{35}{8} \times \frac{1}{5} = \frac{7}{8}$

16. $9\frac{1}{2} \times \frac{1}{4}$ $\frac{19}{2} \times \frac{1}{4} = \frac{19}{8}$ $8\overline{)19} = 2\frac{3}{8}$
$\qquad\qquad\qquad\qquad\qquad\ \ \underline{16}$
$\qquad\qquad\qquad\qquad\qquad\ \ \ 3$

17. $7\frac{1}{4} \times \frac{4}{10}$ $\frac{29}{4} \times \frac{4}{10} = \frac{29}{10} = 2\frac{9}{10}$

18. $12\frac{1}{2} \times \frac{5}{6}$ $\frac{25}{2} \times \frac{5}{6} = \frac{125}{12}$ $12\overline{)125} = 10\frac{5}{12}$
$\qquad\qquad\qquad\qquad\qquad\qquad\qquad \underline{12}$
$\qquad\qquad\qquad\qquad\qquad\qquad\qquad\ \ 5$

19. $21\frac{2}{3} \times \frac{1}{2}$ $\frac{65}{3} \times \frac{1}{2} = \frac{65}{6}$ $6\overline{)65} = 10\frac{5}{6}$
$\qquad\qquad\qquad\qquad\qquad\qquad\quad \underline{6}$
$\qquad\qquad\qquad\qquad\qquad\qquad\quad\ 5$

20. $15\frac{1}{4} \times \frac{3}{5}$ $\frac{61}{4} \times \frac{3}{5} = \frac{183}{20}$ $20\overline{)183} = 9\frac{3}{20}$
$\qquad\qquad\qquad\qquad\qquad\qquad\qquad \underline{160}$
$\qquad\qquad\qquad\qquad\qquad\qquad\qquad\ \ 23$

Passing score is no more than *3* errors.

Section 11   How to Multiply Two Mixed Numbers

Consider the following problem:

$$9\frac{2}{5} \times 7\frac{3}{8}$$

Notice that the problem is to multiply two mixed numbers. Here is all you do.

Problem	Step 1 Change the Mixed Numbers to Improper Fractions
$9\frac{2}{5} \times 7\frac{3}{8}$	$\frac{47}{5} \times \frac{59}{8}$

Step 2 Multiply	Step 3 Change the Result to a Mixed Number
$\frac{47}{5} \times \frac{59}{8} = \frac{2,773}{40}$	$\frac{2,773}{40} = 69\frac{13}{40}$

Look at the above chart.

1. What is the first step?

2. What is the second step?

3. What is the third step?

Let us try several examples. Be sure to follow the step-by-step procedures.

Consider the following problem:

$$10\frac{2}{3} \times 6\frac{1}{2}$$

4. Step 1. Change the mixed numbers to improper fractions.

5. Step 2. Multiply the fractions.

6. Step 3. Change the result to a mixed number.

Solve each of the following problems.

7. $20\frac{1}{3} \times 2\frac{1}{4}$

$\frac{61}{3} \times \frac{\cancel{9}^3}{4} = \frac{183}{4}$

$4\overline{)183} = 45\frac{3}{4}$ $\begin{array}{r} 45 \\ \underline{16} \\ 23 \\ \underline{20} \end{array}$ $\frac{20}{3}$

8. $9\frac{1}{2} \times 4\frac{3}{5}$

$$\frac{19}{2} \times \frac{23}{5} = \frac{437}{10}$$

$$10\overline{)437} = 43\,\tfrac{7}{10}$$

9. $2\frac{3}{4} \times 1\frac{4}{5}$

$$\frac{11}{4} \times \frac{9}{5} = \frac{99}{20}$$

$$20\overline{)99} = 4\tfrac{19}{20}$$

10. $7\frac{1}{2} \times 10\frac{1}{3}$

$$\frac{15}{2} \times \frac{31}{3} = \frac{155}{2}$$

$$2\overline{)155} = 77\tfrac{1}{2}$$

Passing score is no more than *1* error.

Section 12   A Shortcut Method for Multiplying Fractions

Consider the following problem:

$$\frac{3}{4} \times \frac{8}{13} = \frac{24}{52} = \frac{12}{26} = \frac{6}{13}$$

Whenever two fractions are to be multiplied, we multiply their numerators and then their denominators, arriving at a new fraction, which we then try to simplify if we can. Frequently, we are able to simplify some numbers before multiplication by dividing.

For instance, consider

$$\frac{3}{4} \times \frac{8}{13}$$

Notice that the 8 can be divided evenly by 4. Notice the following solution:

$$\frac{3}{\underset{1}{\cancel{4}}} \times \frac{\overset{2}{\cancel{8}}}{13}$$

After simplifying, the fractions are multiplied:

$$\frac{3}{\underset{1}{\cancel{4}}} \times \frac{\overset{2}{\cancel{8}}}{13} = \frac{6}{13}$$

That is all there is to it.

Look at the following problem:

$$\frac{2}{5} \times \frac{10}{7}$$

Notice that the 10 can be divided evenly by 5.

$$\frac{2}{\underset{1}{\cancel{5}}} \times \frac{\overset{2}{\cancel{10}}}{7} = \frac{4}{7}$$

Bear in mind that simplifying makes the multiplication easier.

Look at the following problem:

$$\frac{3}{4} \times \frac{1}{150}$$

Notice that the 150 can be divided evenly by the 3.

$$\frac{\overset{1}{\cancel{3}}}{4} \times \frac{1}{\underset{50}{\cancel{150}}} = \frac{1}{200}$$

Wherever possible, divide before multiplying each of the following fractions:

1. $\dfrac{1}{3} \times \dfrac{9}{12} = \dfrac{1}{4}$

2. $\dfrac{5}{14} \times \dfrac{7}{8} = \dfrac{5}{16}$

3. $\dfrac{3}{7} \times \dfrac{21}{4} = \dfrac{9}{4} = 2\tfrac{1}{4}$

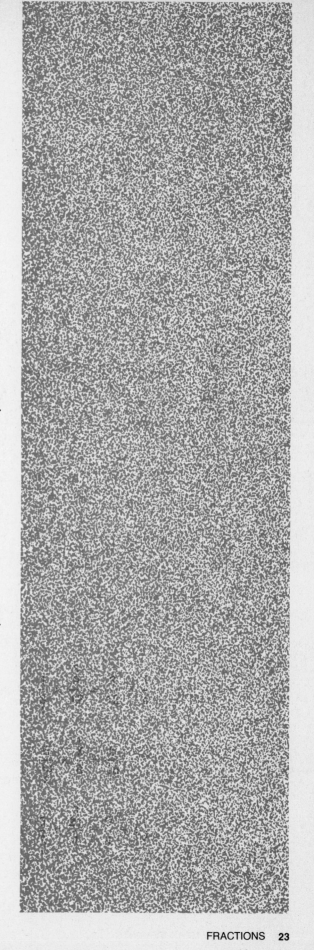

4. $\dfrac{\cancel{7}}{9} \times \dfrac{5}{28} = \dfrac{5}{36}$

5. $\dfrac{6}{11} \times \dfrac{1}{18} = \dfrac{1}{33}$

6. $\dfrac{2}{3} \times \dfrac{27}{5} = \dfrac{18}{5} = 3\tfrac{3}{5}$

7. $\dfrac{4}{7} \times \dfrac{21}{15} = \dfrac{12}{15} = \dfrac{4}{5}$

8. $\dfrac{5}{6} \times \dfrac{30}{20} = \dfrac{15}{12} = 1\tfrac{1}{4}$

9. $\dfrac{5}{20} \times \dfrac{10}{30} = \dfrac{1}{12}$

10. $\dfrac{7}{10} \times \dfrac{20}{35} = \dfrac{2}{5}$

Passing score is no more than *1* error.

Section 13 Dividing Fractions

In order to divide fractions, you must know how to invert fractions.

Read the following:

Fraction	*Inverted Fraction*
$\dfrac{2}{3}$	$\dfrac{3}{2}$

Whenever you invert a fraction, the denominator becomes the numerator, and the numerator becomes the denominator.

Thus, when $\dfrac{2}{3}$ is inverted, it becomes $\dfrac{3}{2}$.

Invert each of the following fractions:

1. $\dfrac{5}{6}$ $\dfrac{6}{5}$

2. $\dfrac{9}{11}$ $\dfrac{11}{9}$

3. $\dfrac{4}{5}$ $\dfrac{5}{4}$

4. $\dfrac{13}{17}$ $\dfrac{17}{13}$

5. $\dfrac{10}{17}$ $\dfrac{17}{10}$

Passing score is *0* errors.

Section 14   How to Divide One Fraction by Another

Consider the following problem:

$$\frac{2}{3} \div \frac{1}{2}$$

Here is all you do.

Problem	Step 1 Invert the Fraction You Are Dividing by
$\dfrac{2}{3} \div \dfrac{1}{2}$	$\dfrac{2}{1}$

Step 2
Multiply the Fractions

$$\frac{2}{3} \times \frac{2}{1} = \frac{4}{3} = 1\frac{1}{3}$$

Look at the above chart.

1. What is the first step?

2. What is the second step?

Let's try several examples.

Consider the following problem:

$$\frac{3}{4} \div \frac{4}{5}$$

3. Invert the fraction you are dividing by.

4. Multiply the fractions. $\frac{15}{16}$

5. $\frac{9}{10} \div \frac{4}{5} = \frac{9}{8} = 1\frac{1}{8}$

6. $\frac{2}{9} \div \frac{4}{11} = \frac{11}{18}$

7. $\frac{3}{4} \div \frac{7}{2} = \frac{3}{14}$

8. $\frac{7}{8} \div \frac{5}{6} = \frac{21}{20} = 1\frac{1}{20}$

9. $\frac{5}{6} \div \frac{20}{24} = 1$

10. $\frac{4}{5} \div \frac{3}{4} = \frac{16}{15} = 1\frac{1}{15}$

Consider the following problem:

$$7\frac{4}{5} \div 2\frac{2}{3}$$

11. Change the mixed numbers to improper fractions.

12. Divide.

13. $1\frac{2}{3} \div 3\frac{1}{2}$ $\frac{5}{3} \times \frac{2}{7} = \frac{10}{21}$

14. $2\frac{3}{4} \div 1\frac{1}{3}$ $\frac{11}{4} \times \frac{3}{4} = \frac{33}{16}$ $16\overline{)33} = 2\frac{1}{16}$

15. $4\frac{1}{4} \div 2\frac{1}{3}$ $\frac{17}{4} \times \frac{3}{7} = \frac{51}{28} = 28\overline{)51} = 1\frac{23}{28}$

16. $5\frac{2}{3} \div 6\frac{1}{8}$ $\frac{17}{3} \times \frac{8}{49} = \frac{136}{147}$

17. $3\frac{1}{5} \div 9\frac{2}{3}$ $\frac{16}{5} \times \frac{3}{29} = \frac{48}{145}$

18. $9\frac{1}{5} \div 3\frac{1}{2}$ $\frac{46}{5} \times \frac{2}{7} = \frac{92}{35}$ $35\overline{)92} = 2\frac{22}{35}$

19. $10\frac{1}{2} \div 1\frac{2}{5}$ $\frac{21}{2} \times \frac{5}{7} = \frac{15}{2} = 7\frac{1}{2}$

20. $8\frac{3}{4} \div 2\frac{5}{8}$ $\frac{35}{4} \times \frac{8}{21} = \frac{10}{3} = 3\frac{1}{3}$

Passing score is no more than *3* errors.

Section 15   Medication Problems

Every tablet contains a certain amount of medication. For instance, a 325-mg aspirin tablet contains 325 mg of aspirin; a 100-mg tablet of ascorbic acid contains 100 mg of ascorbic acid.

Consider the following problem:

A patient has been given two 325-mg aspirin tablets. How much medication has the patient been given?

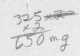

$$\begin{array}{r} 325 \\ \times 2 \\ \hline 650\ mg \end{array}$$

Notice the solution below:

No. of tablets	×	Medication per tablet	=	Total medication
2	×	325 mg	=	650 mg

1. How do you determine the amount of medication the patient was given?

Let's try several problems.

2. A nurse used two 120-mg tablets in the preparation of a medication. How much medication did she use?

120×2 = 240mg

3. During a 24-hour period a patient was given four phenobarbital tablets, 15 mg each. How much phenobarbital did he get?

15 ×4 60mg

Sometimes, you may use less than a whole tablet. For instance, consider the following problem:

If you gave $\frac{1}{2}$ of a 250-mg chlorothiazide tablet, how much drug did you give?

Notice the solution below:

No. of tablets	×	Medication per tablet	=	Total medication
$\frac{1}{2}$	×	250 mg	=	125 mg

Let's try more problems.

4. A patient was given $\frac{1}{2}$ of a $\frac{1}{2}$-gram glutethimide tablet. How much medication did he receive? *¼ gram*

5. If you used $\frac{2}{3}$ of a 300-mg tablet, how much did you use? *$\frac{2}{3}$ × 300mg = 200mg*

6. If you gave $\frac{1}{2}$ of a tablet containing 10 mg oxyphencyclimine HCl and 25 mg hydroxyzine HCl, how much of each medication did you give?

5 mg oxyphencyclimine HCL
12½ mg hydroxyzine HCL

7. If an ampul contains 20 mg of a drug, how much is there in $\frac{3}{4}$ of an ampul? *$\frac{3}{4}$ × 20 = 15mg*

Consider the following problem:

To give 50 mg of ascorbic acid from 100-mg tablets, how many tablets would you use? ½

Notice the solution below:

$$\frac{\text{Total medication}}{\text{Medication per tablet}} = \frac{\text{Number of}}{\text{tablets}}$$

$$\frac{50}{100} = \frac{1}{2} \text{ tablet}$$

Let's try several problems.

8. To give 125 mg tolbutamide from 250-mg tolbutamide tablets, how many tablets would you use? ½

9. To give 50 mg of aminophylline from 100-mg tablets, how many tablets would you use? ½

10. To give $7\frac{1}{2}$ mg of hydrocortisone from 5-mg tablets, how many tablets would you use? 1½

    $\frac{15}{2} \times \frac{1}{5mg} = \frac{3}{2} = 1\frac{1}{2}$

11. To give 6 mg of Myleran from 2-mg tablets, how many tablets would you use?

    $\frac{36mg}{2mg} = 3$

12. To give $\frac{1}{4}$ mg of Haldol from $\frac{1}{2}$-mg tablets, how many tablets would you use?

    $\frac{1}{4} \times \frac{2}{1} = \frac{1}{2}$

13. To give 500 mg of erythromycin from 250-mg tablets, how many tablets would you use? 2

    $\frac{500}{250}$

14. To give 30 mg from 20-mg tablets, how many tablets would you use?

    $\frac{30}{20} = 1\frac{1}{2}$

15. To give 16 mg of codeine sulfate from 32-mg tablets, how many tablets would you use? $\frac{16}{32} = \frac{1}{2}$

16. The doctor orders 45 mg of a medication. If the tablets are 90 mg, how many tablets should be taken?

    $\frac{45}{90} = \frac{1}{2}$

17. A patient took two 15-mg tablets daily for a period of one week. How much medication did he take?

    $2 \times 15mg \times 7 = 210mg$

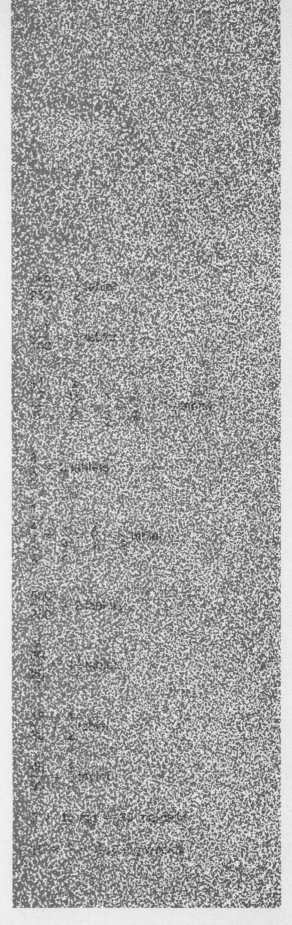

18. If you gave three 45-mg capsules, how much medication did you give?

$3 \times 45 \frac{5}{2} mg = 135 mg$

19. To give 15 mg of warfarin sodium from $7\frac{1}{2}$-mg tablets, how many tablets would you use?

$15 mg \quad \frac{2}{15} = 2$

20. If each ml of an elixir with codeine contains $2\frac{2}{5}$ mg of codeine phosphate, how much codeine phosphate will be present in 5 ml of the elixir?

$5 \times \frac{12}{5} = 12 mg \quad \frac{ml}{ml}$

Passing score is no more than *3* errors.

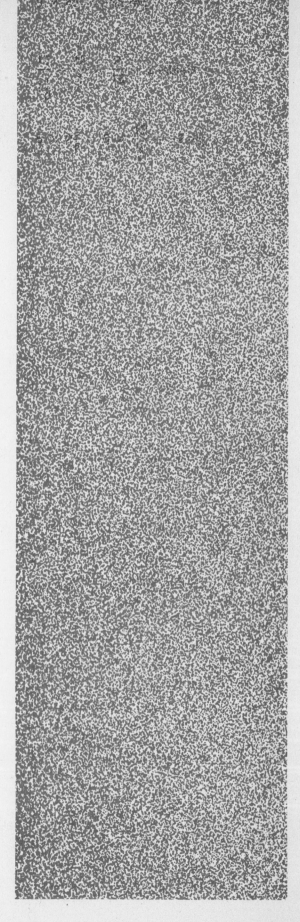

Chapter **2**

Decimals

Section 1   Introduction

In arithmetic, there are two ways of writing *three-tenths*. As a fraction:

$$\frac{3}{10}$$

Or as a decimal:

$$0.3$$

Express each of the following decimals as fractions.

1. 0.2 $\frac{2}{10}$

2. 0.4 $\frac{4}{10}$

3. 0.1 $\frac{1}{10}$

4. 0.5 $\frac{5}{10}$

5. 0.9 $\frac{9}{10}$

6. 0.6 $\frac{6}{10}$

A mixed number may also be expressed as a decimal. For instance:

$$4\frac{1}{10} = 4.1$$

Express each of the following mixed numbers as decimals.

1. $5\frac{2}{10}$ 5.2

2. $4\frac{3}{10}$ 4.3

3. $603\frac{7}{10}$ 603.7

4. $397\frac{4}{10}$ 397.4

Consider the following decimal:

$$2.01$$

Notice that there are two digits to the right of the decimal point. When there are two digits to the right of the decimal point, the decimal is expressed in hundredths.

For instance:

$$2.01 = 2\frac{1}{100}$$

Express each of the following decimals as fractions or mixed numbers.

1. 3.05 $3\frac{5}{100}$

2. 12.68 $12\frac{68}{100}$

3. 0.77 $\frac{77}{100}$

4. 0.80 $\frac{80}{100}$

5. 423.04 $423\frac{4}{100}$

6. 49.31 $49\frac{31}{100}$

7. 23.18 $23\frac{18}{100}$

Consider the following decimal:

$$2.001$$

Notice that there are three digits to the right of the decimal point. When there are three digits to the right of the decimal point, the decimal is expressed in thousandths.

For instance:

$$2.001 = 2\frac{1}{1,000}$$

Express each of the following decimals as mixed numbers.

1. 9.012 $9\frac{12}{1000}$

2. 21.369 $21\frac{369}{1000}$

3. 4.003 $4\frac{3}{1000}$

Consider the following decimal:

$$2.0001$$

Notice that there are four digits to the right of the decimal point. When there are four digits to the right of the decimal point, the decimal is expressed in ten-thousandths. For instance:

$$2.0001 = 2\frac{1}{10,000}$$

Express each of the following decimals as mixed numbers.

1. 2.0195 $2\frac{195}{10000}$

2. 4.0003 $4\frac{3}{10000}$

3. 8.0035 $8\frac{35}{10000}$

4. 11.4122 $11\frac{4122}{10000}$

Change the following fractions and mixed numbers to decimals.

1. $\frac{6}{10}$ .6

2. $3\frac{7}{10}$ 3.7

3. $1\frac{3}{10,000}$ 1.0003

4. $\frac{2}{100}$ .02

5. $\frac{9}{1,000}$ .009

6. $121\frac{5}{100}$ 121.05

7. $13\frac{2}{10}$ 13.2

8. $37\frac{1}{100}$ 37.01

9. $100\frac{2}{1,000}$ 100.002

10. $37\frac{18}{100}$ 37.18

11. $7\frac{4}{1,000}$ 7.004

12. $9\frac{7}{10,000}$ 9.0007

13. $25\frac{16}{100}$ 25.16

14. $71\frac{21}{1,000}$ 71.021

15. $101\frac{83}{100}$ 101.83

16. $63\frac{375}{10,000}$ 63.0375

17. $11\frac{4}{100}$ 11.04

18. $29\frac{67}{1,000}$ 29.067

Passing score is no more than *5* errors.

Section 2   Multiplying Decimals by 10, 100, and 1,000

To multiply a decimal by 10, simply move the decimal point one place to the right. For instance:

$$5.2 \times 10 = 5.2 = 52$$

Notice that when the decimal point is moved one place to the right, 5.2 becomes 52.

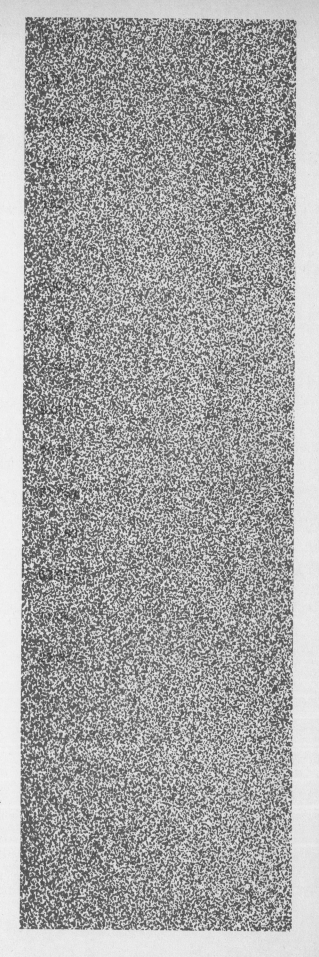

Let's consider another example.

$$4.64 \times 10$$

1. How do you multiply a decimal by 10?

2. Multiply 4.64 by 10. *46.4*

Let's try a few problems.

3. 13.2×10 *132*

4. 37.9×10 *379*

5. 3.05×10 *30.5*

6. 111.2×10 *1112*

7. 11.29×10 *112.9*

8. 10.0×10 *100*

9. 133.6×10 *1336*

10. 0.106×10 *1.06*

To multiply a decimal by 100, move the decimal point two places to the right. For instance:

$$4.64 \times 100 = 4.64 = 464$$

Let's consider another example.

$$5.246 \times 100$$

11. How do you multiply a decimal by 100?

12. Multiply 5.246 by 100. *524.6*

13. 627.81×100 *62781*

14. 1.314×100 *131.4*

15. 39.56×100 *3956*

16. 0.0054×100 *.54*

To multiply a decimal by 1,000, move the decimal point three places to the right. For instance:

$$7.576 \times 1,000 = 7,576$$

17. $1.392 \times 1,000$

1392

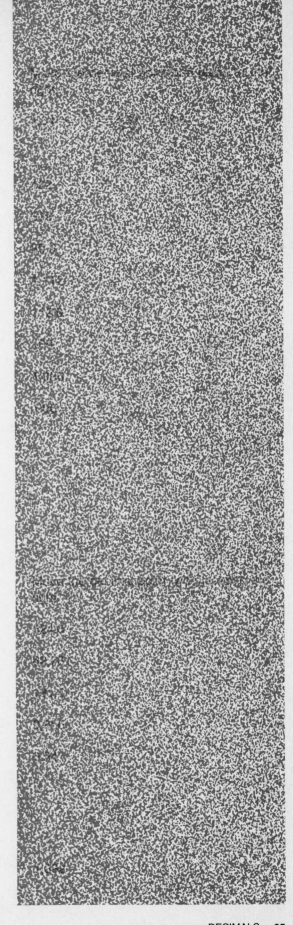

18. 0.0751 × 1,000   *75.1*

19. 18.720 × 1,000   *18720*

20. 173.269 × 1,000   *173269*

21. 100.2978 × 1,000   *100,297.8*

22. 35.06 × 1,000   *35060*

Passing score is no more than *4* errors.

Section 3 Dividing Decimals by 10, 100, and 1,000

To divide a decimal by 10, simply move the decimal point one place to the left. For instance:

$$5.2 \div 10 = 5.2 = 0.52$$

Notice that when the decimal point is moved one place to the left, 5.2 becomes 0.52.

To divide a decimal by 100, move the decimal point two places to the left; to divide by 1,000, move the decimal point three places to the left. For instance:

$$4{,}563.2 \div 100 = 4{,}563.2 = 45.632$$

$$4{,}563.2 \div 1{,}000 = 4{,}563.2 = 4.5632$$

Let us try a few problems.

1. 1,932.66 ÷ 10   *193.266*

2. 237.09 ÷ 100   *2.3709*

3. 789.6 ÷ 1,000   *.7896*

4. 489.29 ÷ 100   *4.8929*

5. 306.2 ÷ 10   *30.62*

6. 0.916 ÷ 100   *.00916*

7. 12.5 ÷ 10   *1.25*

8. 1,143 ÷ 1,000   *1.143*

9. 3,167 ÷ 100   *31.67*

10. 921.2 ÷ 1,000   *.9212*

11. 293.65 ÷ 10   *29.365*

12. 765.3 ÷ 100   *7.653*

Passing score is no more than *2* errors.

Section 4   Changing Decimals to Fractions

Change 0.75 to a fraction.

$$0.75 = \frac{75}{100} = \frac{3}{4}$$

Notice that whenever we change a decimal to a fraction, we always express the fraction in its simplest terms.

Let us try several problems. Change each of the following decimals to fractions.

1. 0.60 $\frac{60}{100} = \frac{3}{5}$

2. 0.25 $\frac{25}{100} = \frac{1}{4}$

3. 0.70 $\frac{70}{100} = \frac{7}{10}$

4. 0.55 $\frac{55}{100} = \frac{11}{20}$

5. 0.20 $\frac{20}{100} = \frac{1}{5}$

6. 0.72 $\frac{72}{100} = \frac{36}{50} = \frac{18}{25}$

7. 0.38 $\frac{38}{100} = \frac{19}{50}$

8. 0.85 $\frac{85}{100} = \frac{17}{20}$

9. 0.22 $\frac{22}{100} = \frac{11}{50}$

10. 0.12 $\frac{12}{100} = \frac{6}{50} = \frac{3}{25}$

11. 0.24 $\frac{24}{100} = \frac{12}{50} = \frac{6}{25}$

12. 0.93 $\frac{93}{100}$

Passing score is no more than *3* errors.

Section 5   Changing Per Cents to Decimals

To change per cents to decimals, move the decimal point two places to the left.

For instance:

$$67\% = 0.67 \left(\text{Bear in mind that } 67\% = \frac{67}{100}. \right)$$
$$87\% = 0.87$$
$$87.6\% = 0.876$$
$$93.69\% = 0.9369$$

Let's try several problems.

Change the following per cents to decimals.

1. 97% .97

2. 37% .37

3. 29.5% .295

4. 11.8% .118

5. 10% .10

6. 22.89% .2289

7. 7.5% .075

8. 1.69% .0169

9. 95.2% .952

10. 28.6% .286

Passing score is no more than *1* error.

Section 6   Changing a Decimal to a Per Cent

To change a decimal to a per cent, move the decimal point two places to the right.

For instance:

$$0.57 = 57\%$$
$$0.62 = 62\%$$
$$0.657 = 65.7\%$$

Let's try several problems.

Change the following decimals to per cents.

1. 0.693   69.3%
2. 2.29   229%
3. 6.4   640%
4. 0.29   29%
5. 0.83   83%
6. 0.09   9%
7. 0.018   1.8%
8. 0.0029   .29%
9. 1.10   110%
10. 0.026   2.6%

Passing score is no more than *1* error.

Section 7   Changing a Per Cent to a Fraction

Here is how to change 20% to a fraction.

$$20\% = \frac{20}{100} = \frac{1}{5}$$

Let's try several problems.

Change the following per cents to fractions.

1. 25% $\frac{25}{100} = \frac{1}{4}$

2. 75% $\frac{75}{100} = \frac{3}{4}$

3. 70% $\frac{70}{100} = \frac{7}{10}$

4. 60% $\frac{60}{100} = \frac{3}{5}$

5. 45% $\frac{45}{100} = \frac{9}{20}$

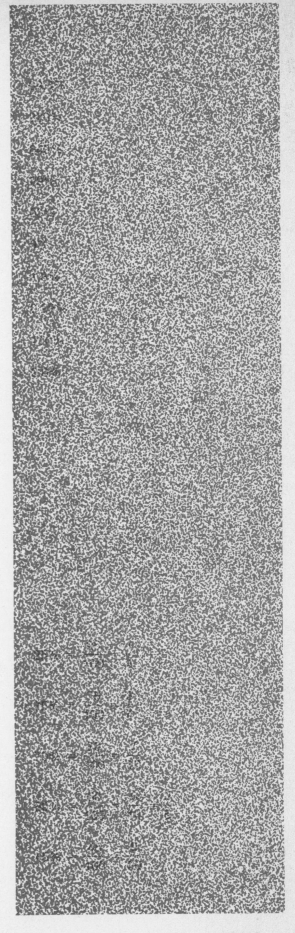

6. 63% $\frac{63}{100}$

7. 22% $\frac{22}{100} = \frac{11}{50}$

8. 29% $\frac{29}{100}$

9. 64% $\frac{64}{100} = \frac{32}{50} = \frac{16}{25}$

10. 48% $\frac{48}{100} = \frac{24}{50} = \frac{12}{25}$

Passing score is no more than *1* error.

Section 8   Changing Fractions to Decimals

Any fraction represents one number divided by another. For instance, $\frac{3}{4}$ represents $3 \div 4$; $\frac{5}{7}$ represents $5 \div 7$.

To change a fraction to a decimal, simply divide the numerator by the denominator.

Problem	Step 1	Step 2
Change $\frac{3}{4}$ to a decimal	Indicate the decimal point for the result $\overset{.}{4\overline{)3.00}}$	Divide $\begin{array}{r} 0.75 \\ 4\overline{)3.00} \\ \underline{2\,8} \\ 20 \\ \underline{20} \end{array}$

Notice Step 1. *It is important to indicate the decimal point before you begin to divide.*

Change the following fractions to decimals.

1. $\frac{1}{2}$ .5

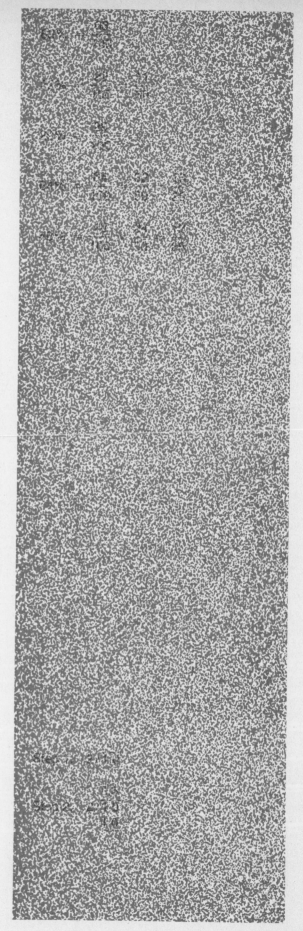

2. $\frac{1}{4}$

$$4\overline{)1.00} \quad .25$$
$$\underline{8}$$
$$20$$

3. $\frac{2}{3}$

$$3\overline{)2.00} \quad .66$$
$$\underline{18}$$
$$20$$
$$\underline{18}$$
$$2$$

4. $\frac{16}{25}$

$$25\overline{)16.00} \quad .64$$
$$\underline{150}$$
$$100$$
$$\underline{100}$$

5. $\frac{11}{50}$

$$50\overline{)11.00} \quad .22$$
$$\underline{100}$$
$$100$$
$$\underline{100}$$

6. $\frac{9}{20}$

$$20\overline{)9.00} \quad .45$$
$$\underline{80}$$
$$100$$
$$\underline{100}$$

7. $\frac{17}{50}$

$$50\overline{)17.00} \quad \frac{.34}{}$$
$$\quad \underline{150}$$
$$\quad 200$$

8. $\frac{9}{25}$

$$25\overline{)9.00} \quad \frac{.36}{}$$
$$\quad \underline{75}$$
$$\quad 150$$
$$\quad 150$$

9. $\frac{2}{5}$

$$5\overline{)2.00} \quad \frac{.4}{}$$
$$\quad 20$$

10. $\frac{1}{8}$

$$8\overline{)1.000} \quad \frac{.125}{}$$
$$\quad \underline{8}$$
$$\quad 20$$
$$\quad 16$$
$$\quad 40$$
$$\quad 40$$

Passing score is no more than *2* errors.

Section 9   Multiplying by a Per Cent

One way to multiply by a per cent is to change the per cent to a fraction. For instance:

Problem

What is 25% of 176?

Step 1	Step 2
$25\% = \dfrac{25}{100} = \dfrac{1}{4}$	$\dfrac{1}{4} \times 176 = \dfrac{176}{4} = 44$

A second way is to change the per cent to a decimal. For instance:

Problem

What is 25% of 176?

Step 1	Step 2
$25\% = 0.25$	$0.25 \times 176 = 44$

Note: Bear in mind that "of" usually means multiply.

Solve each of the following problems two ways.

1. 25% of 250

$$\frac{25}{100} = \frac{1}{4} \times \frac{250}{1} = 4\overline{)250.1} \quad \begin{array}{r} 62.5 \\ \underline{24} \\ 10 \\ \underline{9} \\ 20 \end{array}$$

$$.25 \times 250 = 62.5$$

2. 50% of 640

$$\frac{50}{100} = \frac{1}{2} \times \frac{640}{1} = 320$$

$$.50 \times 100 = 320$$

3. 75% of 1,000

$$\frac{75}{100} = \frac{3}{4} \times \frac{1000}{1} = 4\overline{)3000} \quad \begin{array}{r} 250 \\ \underline{30} \\ 20 \end{array}$$

$$.75 \times 1000 = 750$$

4. 30% of 420

$$\frac{30}{100} = \frac{3}{10} \times \frac{420}{1} = 126$$

$$.30 \times 420 = 126$$

5. 10% of 90

$$\frac{10}{100} = \frac{1}{10} \times \frac{90}{1} = 9$$

$$.1 \times 90 = 9$$

6. 95% of 400

$$\frac{95}{100} = \frac{19}{20} \times \frac{400}{1} = 380$$

$$.95 \times 400 = 380$$

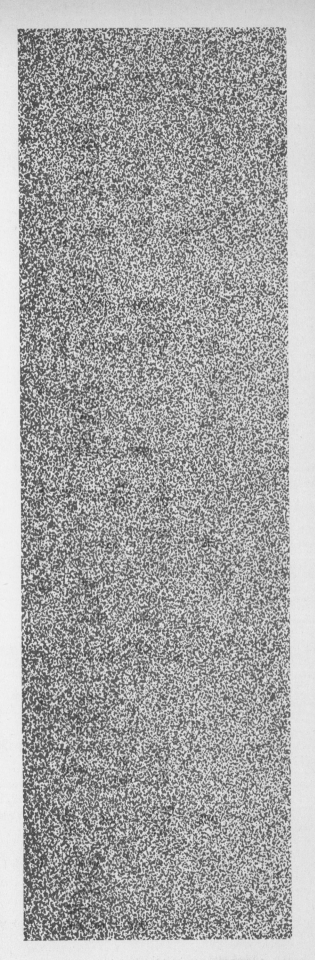

7. 25% of 800

$$\frac{25}{100} = \frac{1}{\cancel{4}} \times \frac{\cancel{800}^{200}}{1} = 200$$

$.25 \times 800 = 200$

8. 42% of 800

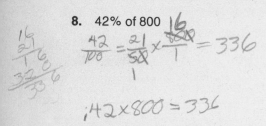

$$\frac{42}{100} = \frac{21}{\cancel{50}} \times \frac{\cancel{800}^{16}}{1} = 336$$

$.42 \times 800 = 336$

9. 40% of 1,000

$$\frac{4\cancel{0}}{10\cancel{0}} = \frac{2}{5} \times \frac{\cancel{1000}^{200}}{1} = 400$$

$.40 \times 1000 = 400$

10. 28% of 600

$$\frac{28}{100} = \frac{14}{50} = \frac{7}{\cancel{25}} \times \frac{\cancel{600}^{24}}{1} = 168$$

$.28 \times 600 = 168$

Passing score is no more than *2* errors.

Section 10   Multiplying and Dividing Decimals by Whole Numbers

Multiplying decimals is the same as multiplying whole numbers except that you must be careful to put the decimal point in the proper place.

Let's consider where to put the decimal point.

Look at the following problem:

$$25.678 \times 16{,}076 = 412799528$$

1. How many digits are to the right of the decimal point of 25.678?   *3*

2. What is the third digit from the right in the answer?   *5*

Copy 412799528 on a piece of paper.

3. Now place the decimal point before the third digit from the right.   *412799.528*

That's all there is to it.

Let us try a few more examples of putting the decimal point in the proper place.

$$2.35 \times 450 = 1057{,}50$$

4. Count the digits to the right of the decimal point.

5. What is the second digit from the right in the answer?

6. Place the decimal point before the second digit from the right in the answer.

Notice the following example:

$$5.7 \times 67 = 381{,}9$$

7. How many digits are to the right of the decimal point?   \

8. Place the decimal point in its proper place in the answer.

$$0.234 \times 6 = 1{,}404$$

9. How many digits are to the right of the decimal point?

10. Place the decimal point in its proper place in the answer.

Indicate the decimal point in each of the following answers.

11. $1.6 \times 25 = 400$ *40.0*

12. $29.1 \times 10 = 2910$ *291.0*

13. $164 \times 0.2 = 328$ *32.8*

14. $253 \times 1.5 = 3795$ *379.5*

15. $1.15 \times 200 = 23000$ *230.00*

16. $115 \times 0.5 = 575$ *57.5*

17. $240 \times 2.8 = 6720$ *672.0*

18. $750 \times 10.21 = 7657{,}50$ *7657.50*

19. $2.3 \times 9{,}000 = 207000$

20. $4.6 \times 450 = 20700$

Passing score is no more than *3* errors.

Section 11 Multiplying Two Decimals

When multiplying two decimals, we must be careful to put the decimal point in its proper place.

Let us consider where to put the decimal point.

Look at the following problem:

$$25.678 \times 160.76 = 412799528$$

1. How many digits are to the right of the decimal point in 25.678?

2. How many digits are to the right of the decimal point in 160.76?

When multiplying two decimals, add the number of digits to the right of each decimal point.

In the above example, there is a total of two + three, or five, digits to the right of the two decimal points.

3. Now place the decimal point before the fifth digit from the right in the answer.

That's all there is to it.

Indicate where to put the decimal point in each of the following examples.

4. $10.5 \times 1.5 = 1575$

5. $10.5 \times 0.2 = 210$

6. $0.6 \times 30.5 = 1830$

7. $7.2 \times 0.1 = 72$

8. $2.4 \times 1.4 = 336$

9. $191.4 \times 0.4 = 7656$

10. $0.5 \times 200.5 = 10025$

11. $0.2 \times 2.0 = 40$

12. $1.2 \times 6.22 = 7464$

13. $10.2 \times 10.22 = 104244$

14. $1.21 \times 6.2 = 7502$

15. $1.5 \times 1000.8 = 150120$

Passing score is no more than *2* errors.

Consider the following problem:

$$0.404 \times 0.162 = 65448$$

16. What is the total number of digits to the right of the decimal points?

17. How many digits *must* appear to the right of the decimal point in the answer?

However, there are only five digits in the answer. Therefore, notice the answer below:

$$0.065448$$

Whenever the answer does not have enough digits, add as many zeros as are needed to the *left* of the digits.

Let's try several additional problems.

18. $0.902 \times 0.100 = 90200$ .090200

19. $0.700 \times 0.115 = 80500$ .080500

20. $0.240 \times 0.404 = 96960$ .096960

21. $0.122 \times 0.200 = 24400$ .024400

22. $0.525 \times 0.220 = 115500$ .115500

Passing score is no more than *2* errors.

Section 12   Medication Problems

1. If you gave 20% of a 30-mg tablet, how much medication did you give?

$$\frac{20}{100} = \frac{1}{5} \times \frac{30}{1} = 6 \, mg$$

2. If you gave 50% of a 0.40-gram tablet, how much medication did you give?

$$\frac{50}{100} = \frac{1}{2} \times \frac{40}{1} = .20 \, gram$$

3. If you need 0.10% of 1,000 ml, how much medication do you need?

$$\frac{}{} \times \frac{1000 \, ml}{} = 10 \, ml$$

$\times 1000$
.0010
1.0000

4. If you gave 75% of a 20-ml ampul, how much did you give?  $\frac{75}{100} = \frac{3}{4} \times \frac{20\,ml}{1} = 15ml$

5. What is 50% of 0.050?

$$\begin{array}{r} .50 \\ \times .050 \\ \hline .02500 \end{array}$$

6. What is $\frac{1}{2}$ % of 0.020?

$$\begin{array}{r} .005 \\ \times .020 \\ \hline .000100 \end{array}$$

7. What is 62.5% of 560?

$$\begin{array}{r} .625 \\ \times 560 \\ \hline 37500 \\ 3125000 \\ \hline 350.000 \end{array}$$

8. If you need 5% of a 60-mg tablet, how much do you need?

$$\begin{array}{r} .05 \\ \times 60 \\ \hline 3.00 \end{array}$$

Passing score is *0* errors.

Chapter 3

Temperature Conversion

Section 1 Changing from Celsius to Fahrenheit

We are all familiar with the Fahrenheit (F) temperature scale because it is used on household as well as clinical thermometers. However, European hospitals and an ever-increasing number of American hospitals use the Celsius (C) scale. In some books you may see the term "Celsius (C) temperature" and in others "centigrade (C) temperature." Both these terms may be used interchangeably.

Look at the illustration on the next page.

A patient's temperature was taken with a Fahrenheit as well as a Celsius thermometer.

1. What was his temperature according to the Celsius scale?

2. What was his temperature according to the Fahrenheit scale?

Sometimes, you may take a patient's temperature using a Celsius thermometer. However, it may be necessary to report the temperature according to the Fahrenheit scale. For this reason, a nurse must know how to convert a Celsius reading to a Fahrenheit reading.

On the other hand, you may take the patient's temperature using a Fahrenheit thermometer and be required to make the report according to the Celsius scale. Therefore, it is necessary to know how to convert Fahrenheit to Celsius.

Now let us find out how to convert a Celsius reading to Fahrenheit. The equation to use is:

$$\text{Fahrenheit reading} = \frac{9}{5} \text{ Celsius reading} + 32°$$

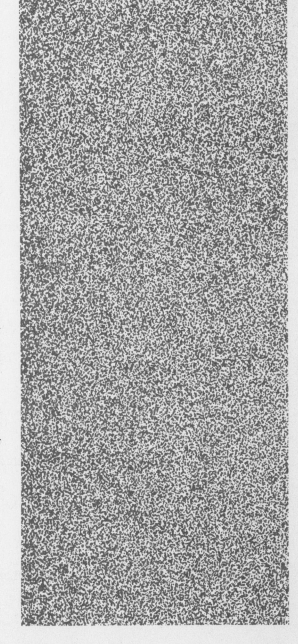

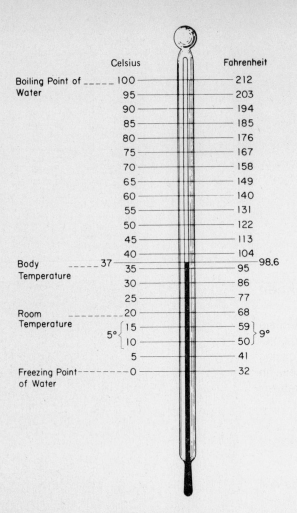

Celsius | Fahrenheit

Boiling Point of ------ 100 ------ 212
Water
95 ------ 203
90 ------ 194
85 ------ 185
80 ------ 176
75 ------ 167
70 ------ 158
65 ------ 149
60 ------ 140
55 ------ 131
50 ------ 122
45 ------ 113
40 ------ 104
Body ----- 37 ------ 98.6
Temperature 35 ------ 95
30 ------ 86
25 ------ 77
Room --------- 20 ------ 68
Temperature 15 ------ 59
5° { 15 ------ 59 } 9°
   { 10 ------ 50 }
5 ------ 41
Freezing Point -------- 0 ------ 32
of Water

If the reading on the Celsius scale is 50°, here is the way to use the equation to determine the Fahrenheit reading.

$$F = \frac{9}{5}C + 32°$$

$$F = \frac{9}{5} \times 50 + 32°$$

$$F = 90 + 32$$

$$F = 122°$$

Now let us try a few problems.

3. If the temperature is 35°C, what is the Fahrenheit reading?

$$\frac{9}{5} \times \frac{35}{1} = 63 + 32 = 95°F$$

4. If the temperature is 39°C, what is the Fahrenheit reading?

$$\frac{9}{5} \times \frac{39}{1} = \frac{351}{5} + 32 = 102.2°F$$

5. If the temperature is 36.8°C, what is the Fahrenheit reading?

$$\frac{9}{5} \times \frac{36.8}{1} = \frac{66.24}{331.20} + 32 = 98.24°$$

6. If the temperature is 40°C, what is the Fahrenheit reading?

$$\frac{9}{5} \times \frac{40}{1} = 72 + 32 = 104°$$

7. If the temperature is 37.8°C, what is the Fahrenheit reading?

$$\frac{9}{5} \times \frac{37.8}{1} = 5\overline{)340.2} = 68.0 + 32 = 100°$$

8. If the temperature is 39.8°C, what is the Fahrenheit reading?

$$\frac{9}{5} \times \frac{39.8}{1} = 5\overline{)358.2} = 71.6 + 32 = 103.6°$$

9. Convert 40.8°C to Fahrenheit.

$$\frac{9}{5} \times \frac{40.8}{1} = 5\overline{)367.2} = 73.4 + 32 = 105.4°$$

10. Convert 38°C to Fahrenheit.

$$\frac{9}{5} \times \frac{38}{1} = 5\overline{)342.0} = 68.4 + 32 = 100.4°$$

11. Convert 38.8°C to Fahrenheit.

$$\frac{9}{5} \times \frac{38.8}{1} = 5\overline{)349.2} = 69.8 + 32 = 101.8°$$

12. Convert 37°C to Fahrenheit.

$$\frac{9}{5} \times \frac{37}{1} = 5\overline{)333} = 66.6 + 32 = 98.6°$$

Passing score is no more than *3* errors.

Section 2   Changing from Fahrenheit to Celsius

The equation to use is:

$$\text{Celsius reading} = \frac{5}{9}(\text{Fahrenheit reading} - 32°)$$

$$C = \frac{5}{9}(F - 32°)$$

If the reading on the Fahrenheit scale is 212°, here's how to determine the reading on the Celsius scale.

$$C = \frac{5}{9}(F - 32°)$$

Step 1. $C = \frac{5}{9}(212 - 32)$

$$C = \frac{5}{9}(180)$$

Step 2. $C = 100°$

Look again at Step 1.

Notice that *before* we multiply, 32° must be subtracted from the Fahrenheit reading.

Now let's try several problems.

1. Convert 104°F to Celsius.

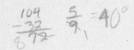

2. Convert 102.9°F to Celsius.

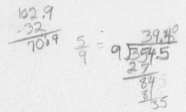

3. Convert 100.4°F to Celsius.

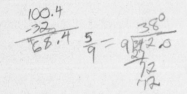

4. Convert 98.2°F to Celsius.

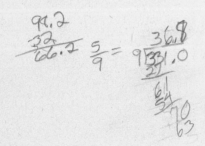

5. Convert 102.2°F to Celsius.

$$\begin{array}{r} 102.2 \\ -32 \\ \hline 70.2 \end{array} \quad \frac{5}{9} = 9\overline{)351.\cancel{8}} \quad \begin{array}{r} 39° \\ 27 \\ \hline 81 \end{array}$$

6. Convert 99.7°F to Celsius.

$$\begin{array}{r} 99.7 \\ -32 \\ \hline 67.7 \end{array} \quad \frac{5}{9} = 9\overline{)338.5}$$

7. Convert 99°F to Celsius.

$$\begin{array}{r} 99 \\ -32 \\ \hline 67 \end{array} \quad \frac{5}{9} = 9\overline{)335.0} \quad \begin{array}{r} 37.2 \\ 27 \\ \hline 65 \\ 63 \\ \hline 20 \end{array}$$

8. Convert 105.8°F to Celsius.

$$\begin{array}{r} 105.8 \\ -32 \\ \hline 73.8 \end{array} \quad \frac{5}{9} = 9\overline{)369.0} \quad \begin{array}{r} 41° \\ 36 \end{array}$$

9. Convert 96.8°F to Celsius.

$$\begin{array}{r} 96.8 \\ -32 \\ \hline 64.8 \end{array} \quad \frac{5}{9} = 9\overline{)324.0} \quad \begin{array}{r} 36° \\ 27 \\ \hline 54 \\ 54 \end{array}$$

10. Convert 98.6°F to Celsius.

$$\begin{array}{r} 98.6 \\ -32 \\ \hline 66.6 \end{array} \quad \frac{5}{9} = 9\overline{)333.0} \quad \begin{array}{r} 37° \\ 27 \\ \hline 63 \\ 63 \end{array}$$

One important fact to remember is that normal body temperature is 98.6°F or 37°C. If you know that a temperature slightly above normal on the Fahrenheit scale should be slightly above 37° on the Celsius scale, you can check to see whether the answer is reasonable.

Passing score is no more than *2* errors.

Chapter 4

The Metric System

Under the English system of measurement, length is measured in yards, feet, and inches; weight is measured in ounces and pounds; and volume is measured in pints, quarts, and gallons.

The metric system is another system of measurement that is used in all scientific work, including medicine.

Section 1   The Measurement of Length in the Metric System

Let us begin by considering the units in which length is measured in the metric system.

The unit of length is the *meter.* (Note: One meter is a little longer than one yard.)

Read the following:

It is 20 kilometers to Paris.

"Kilo" is a prefix that means 1,000. Therefore, a kilometer is 1,000 meters.

1. How many meters are 2 kilometers? 2000

2. How many meters are 5 kilometers? 5000

m is the abbreviation for meters; k is the abbreviation for kilo; therefore, km is the abbreviation for kilometers.*

3. How many meters are 14 km? 14000

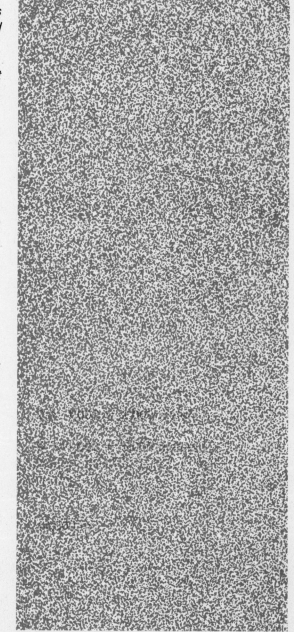

* Kilometers may also be abbreviated as Km. Computers frequently capitalize all letters, so kilometers may also be abbreviated as KM, and meters may also be abbreviated as M.

4. How many meters are 22 km? *22,000*

5. How many meters are 11 km? *11,000*

6. How many meters are 5 km? *5,000*

Consider the following problem:

Problem	Solution
How many kilometers are in 5,435 m?	$\dfrac{5,435}{1,000} = 5.435$ km

To change meters to kilometers, divide by 1,000. (Note: To divide by 1,000, move the decimal point three places to the left.)

Let us try several additional problems.

7. How many kilometers are in 2,800 m? *2.8*

8. How many kilometers are in 7,900 m? *7.9*

9. How many kilometers are in 25,000 m? *25*

10. How many kilometers are in 46,000 m? *46*

11. How many kilometers are in 100,000 m? *100*

12. How many kilometers are in 329,000 m? *329*

13. How many kilometers are in 200,000 m? *200*

14. How many kilometers are in 320 m? *.320*

Consider the following problem:

Problem	Solution
How many meters are in 5.43 km?	$5.43 \times 1,000 = 5,430$ m

To change kilometers to meters, multiply by 1,000. (Note: To multiply by 1,000, move the decimal point three places to the right.)

Let us try some additional problems.

15. How many meters are in 12 km? *12,000*

16. How many meters are in 91.4 km? *91,400*

17. How many meters are in 20.4 km? *20,400*

18. How many meters are in 70.5 km? 70500

19. How many meters are in 0.5 km? 500

20. How many meters are in 0.82 km? 820

Passing score is no more than *4* errors.

Section 2   Centimeters

Read the following:

This shelf is 50 centimeters wide.

"Centi" is a prefix that means one-hundredth. Therefore, a centimeter is one-hundredth of a meter. The abbreviation for centimeter is cm.*

Consider the following problem:

Problem	Solution
How many centimeters are in 5.435 m?	**5.435 × 100 = 543.5 cm**

To change meters to centimeters, multiply by 100. (Note: To multiply by 100, move the decimal point two places to the right.)

Let's try several problems.

1. How many centimeters are in 19.2 m? 1920

2. How many centimeters are in 11 m? 1100

3. How many centimeters are in 35.6 m? 3560

4. How many centimeters are in 21.3 m? 2130

5. How many centimeters are in 95.8 m? 9580

6. How many centimeters are in 33 m? 3300

7. How many centimeters are in 54 m? 5400

8. How many centimeters are in 150 m? 15000

9. How many centimeters are in 87.3 m? 8730

10. How many centimeters are in 299.3 m? 29930

---

* Computers frequently capitalize all letters, so centimeters may also be abbreviated as CM.

Consider the following problem:

Problem	Solution
How many meters are in 5,436.7 cm?	$\dfrac{5,436.7}{100} = 54.367$ m

To change centimeters to meters, divide by 100. (Note: To divide by 100, move the decimal point two places to the left.)

Here are some additional problems.

11. How many meters are in 2,500 cm? 25

12. How many meters are in 18,000 cm? 180

13. How many meters are in 383,000 cm? 3830

14. How many meters are in 21,300 cm? 213

15. How many meters are in 9,580 cm? 95.8

16. How many meters are in 1,500 cm? 15

17. How many meters are in 50 cm? .50

18. How many meters are in 35.1 cm? .351

Passing score is no more than *3* errors.

Section 3   Millimeters

Read the following:

The base of an ampul is 22 millimeters in diameter.

"Milli" is a prefix that means one-thousandth. Therefore, a millimeter is one-thousandth of a meter.

Consider the following problem:

Problem	Solution
How many millimeters are in 0.4563 m?	$0.4563 \times 1,000 = 456.3$ mm

To change meters to millimeters, multiply by 1,000.

The abbreviation for millimeters is mm.*

---

* Computers frequently capitalize all letters, so millimeters may be abbreviated as MM.

Now let us try several problems.

1. How many millimeters are in 0.575 m? *575*

2. How many millimeters are in 35 m? *35000*

3. How many millimeters are in 33.9 m? *33900*

4. How many millimeters are in 6.7 m? *6700*

5. How many millimeters are in 1.9 m? *1900*

6. How many millimeters are in 0.4 m? *400*

7. How many millimeters are in 10.2 m? *10200*

8. How many millimeters are in 1.04 m? *1040*

9. How many millimeters are in 22.1 m? *22100*

10. How many millimeters are in 0.037 m? *37*

Consider the following problem:

Problem	Solution
How many meters are in 5,437.8 mm?	$5,437.8 \div 1,000 = 5.4378$ m

To change millimeters to meters, divide by 1,000.

Here are some additional problems.

11. How many meters are in 22,100 mm? *22.1*

12. How many meters are in 33,900 mm? *33.9*

13. How many meters are in 1,620 mm? *1.62*

14. How many meters are in 620 mm? *.620*

15. How many meters are in 4,600 mm? *4.6*

Passing score is no more than *2* errors.

Section 4 Review

Bear in mind that in going from a large unit to a smaller one, multiply; in going from a small unit to a larger one, divide.

Here are additional practice problems.

1. How many kilometers are in 3,200 m? *3.2*

2. How many meters are in 88 km? *88000*

3. How many centimeters are in 139 m? *13900*

4. How many meters are in 25,300 cm? *253.*

5. How many millimeters are in 1.36 m? *1360*

6. How many meters are in 27,500 mm? *27.5*

7. How many kilometers are in 18,400 m? *18.4*

8. How many meters are in 3.25 km? *3250*

9. How many centimeters are in 127 m? *12700*

10. How many meters are in 16,200 cm? *162*

11. How many kilometers are in 3,050 m? *3.05*

12. How many meters are in 23 km? *23000*

13. How many centimeters are in 361.4 m? *36140*

14. How many meters are in 3,350 cm? *33.5*

15. How many millimeters are in 234 m? *234,000*

16. How many meters are in 7,400 mm? *7.4*

17. How many kilometers are in 185,000 m? *185*

18. How many centimeters are in 24.9 m? *2490*

19. How many millimeters are in 36.1 m? *36100*

20. How many meters are in 47,000 mm? *47*

Passing score is no more than *4* errors.

Section 5   The Measurement of Weight in the Metric System

Read the following:

The book weighs 50 grams.

In the metric system, weight is measured in grams. (Note: One gram is about one-thirtieth of an ounce.)

kg is the abbreviation for kilogram; g is the abbreviation for gram; cg is the abbreviation for centigram; and mg is the abbreviation for milligram.*

Answer the following questions:

1. How many grams are in 1 kg? *1000*

2. What is the abbreviation for a kilogram? *kg*

3. How many grams are in a centigram? *.01 or 1/100*

4. What is the abbreviation for centigram? *cg*

5. How many grams are in a milligram? *1/1000*

6. What is the abbreviation for milligram? *mg*

7. What is the abbreviation for gram? *g*

Now let's try several problems.

8. Change 205 g to kilograms. *.205*

9. How do you change grams to kilograms? *÷ by 1000*

10. Change 5.43 kg to grams. *5430*

11. How do you change kilograms to grams? *x by 1000*

12. How many centigrams are in 5.435 g? *543.5*

13. How do you change grams to centigrams? *x by 100*

14. How many grams are in 5,436.7 cg? *54.367*

15. How do you change centigrams to grams? *÷ by 100*

16. How many milligrams are in 0.3789 g? *378.9*

17. How do you change grams to milligrams? *x by 1000*

18. How many grams are in 5,437.8 mg? *5.4378*

19. How do you change milligrams to grams? *÷ by 1000*

20. How many kilograms are in 56,800 g? *56.8*

21. How many centigrams are in 903 g? *90300*

* In many nursing and nutrition textbooks gram is also abbreviated as Gm or gm. Computers frequently capitalize all letters, so gram may be abbreviated as G, centigram as CG, and milligram as MG.

22. How many grams are in 29,050 cg? 290.5

23. How many milligrams are in 572.8 g? 572,800

24. How many grams are in 17,000 mg? 17

25. How many grams are in 47,100 kg? 47,100,000

26. How many grams are in 93,000 mg? 93

27. How many kilograms are in 237,000 g? 237

28. How many centigrams are in 926.2 g? 92,620

29. How many grams are in 1,936 cg? 19.36

30. How many kilograms are in 705 g? .705

31. How many centigrams are in 48 g? 4,800

32. How many grams are in 2,900 cg? 29

33. How many milligrams are in 135 g? 135,000

34. How many grams are in 58,000 mg? 58

35. How many kilograms are in 75,400 g? 75.4

Passing score is no more than *6* errors. —1

Section 6 The Measurement of Small Weights in the Metric System

An increasing number of medications are becoming available in smaller and smaller amounts. For instance, some medications are measured in micrograms, which is only one-millionth of a gram.

One of the advantages of expressing the weight of a medication in micrograms is that you can use whole numbers. That isn't always true when you are describing small weights in milligrams.

For instance, a medication might be said to weigh 0.05 milligrams. 0.05 milligrams is equal to 50 micrograms. Expressing small weights in micrograms is easier because you can use whole numbers.

Because more and more medications are being measured in micrograms, one of the things you need to be able to do is to convert milligrams to micrograms. It's easy. Keep in mind that 1 milligram is equal to 1,000 micrograms. Therefore, you can change milligrams to micrograms by multiplying the number of milligrams by 1,000. For example:

0.05 milligrams × 1,000 = 50 micrograms

As you have already learned, the abbreviation for milligram is mg (or MG). The abbreviation for microgram is mcg (or MCG).

Try to answer the following questions.

1. How many milligrams are in a gram? *1000*

2. How many micrograms are in a gram? *1000000*

3. How many micrograms are in a milligram? *1100*

4. What's the abbreviation for milligram? *mg*

5. What's the abbreviation for microgram? *mcg*

6. How would you change milligrams to micrograms? *× by 1000*

7. Change 0.05 milligrams to micrograms. *50*

8. Change 0.75 milligrams to micrograms. *750*

On occasion, you may have to change micrograms to milligrams. Once again, that's easy. To change micrograms to milligrams, just divide the number of micrograms by 1,000. For example:

250 micrograms ÷ 1,000 = 0.25 milligrams

9. Change 150 mcg to mg. *.15*

10. Change 75 mcg to mg. *.075*

11. Change 0.2 mg to mcg. *200*

12. Change 0.08 mg to mcg. *80*

13. Change 3 mcg to mg. *.003*

14. Change 0.001 mg to mcg. *1*

15. Change 250 mcg to mg. *.25*

Passing score is no more than *1* error.

Section 7 The Measurement of Volume in the Metric System

Read the following:

I want one liter of milk.

In the metric system, volume is measured in liters. (Note: One liter is about one quart.)

The word liter* is frequently written out, while the word milliliter is abbreviated as ml or ML. In this manual we will always write out the word liter.

Answer the following questions.

1. How many milliliters is 1 liter? *1000*

2. How many liters is 1 ml? *.001 or 1/1000*

3. What is the abbreviation for milliliter? *ml*

Now let's try several problems.

4. How many milliliters are in 2.057 liters? *2057*

5. How do you change liters to milliliters? *× by 1000*

6. How many liters are in 3,759 ml? *3.759*

7. How do you change milliliters to liters? *÷ by 1000*

8. How many liters are in 79,200 ml? *79.2*

9. How many milliliters are in 59.2 liters? *59200*

10. How many liters are in 39,000 ml? *39*

11. How many milliliters are in 0.65 liter? *650*

12. How many liters are in 187 ml? *.187*

13. How many milliliters are in 91.72 liters? *91,720*

Read the following:

I need a cubic centimeter of water.

In the metric system, volume is also measured in cubic centimeters; cm³ or cc† is the abbreviation for cubic centimeters, and one cubic centimeter equals one milliliter.

---

* Liter can be abbreviated as l or L.
† The term cm³ is used by chemists; the term cc is in common medical use.

Let's try a few problems.

14. How many milliliters are in 100 cc? *100*

15. How many cubic centimeters are in 425 ml? *425*

16. How many liters are in 380 cc? *.38*

17. How many cubic centimeters are in 209 ml? *209*

18. How many liters are in 62,843 cc? *62.843*

19. How many cubic centimeters are in 36.4 ml? *36.4*

20. How many cubic centimeters are in 20 liters? *20,000*

21. How many milliliters are in 790 cc? *790*

22. How many liters are in 220 cc? *.22*

23. How many milliliters are in 3,820 cc? *3,820*

Passing score is no more than *5* errors.

Section 8   Review

1. 20 g = *20,000* mg

2. 250 cc = *.25* liter

3. 0.047 m = *47* mm

4. 94.2 cm = *.942* m

5. 200 mcg = *.2* mg

6. 3.08 cc = *3.08* ml

7. 186 mg = *.186* g

8. 0.0058 km = *5.8* m

9. 80 ml = *.08* liter

10. 1.02 liters = *1020* cc

11. 0.075 mg = *75* mcg

12. 0.0516 g = *51.6* mg

13. 47.36 cc = *.04736* liter

14. 6.51 m = <u>6510</u> mm

15. 0.69 g = <u>69</u> cg

16. 78.5 m = <u>7850</u> cm

17. 6 mcg = <u>.006</u> mg

18. 0.0098 liter = <u>9.8</u> ml

19. 8.92 cm = <u>.0892</u> m

20. 0.057 cc = <u>.057</u> ml

21. 91.7 g = <u>91,200</u> kg

22. 0.02 mg = <u>20</u> mcg

23. 0.36 cg = <u>.0036</u> g

24. 381 m = <u>.381</u> km

25. 82.6 mm = <u>.0826</u> m

26. 5.09 mg = <u>.00509</u> g

27. 617 mm = <u>.617</u> m

28. 0.514 kg = <u>514</u> g

29. 0.05 mg = <u>50</u> mcg

30. 28.69 ml = <u>28.69</u> cc

31. 0.005 m = <u>.000005</u> km

32. 45.976 mm = <u>.045976</u> m

33. 8.107 g = <u>8107</u> mg

34. 250 liters = <u>250,000</u> ml

35. 0.000018 km = <u>.018</u> m

36. 3,725 g = <u>3.725</u> kg

37. 90.78 ml = <u>.09078</u> liter

38. 40 mcg = <u>.04</u> mg

39. 54.3 cg = <u>.543</u> g

40. 9.36 liters = <u>9360</u> cc

41. 0.009625 kg = <u>9.625</u> g

42. 429 ml = _429_ cc

43. 0.016 g = _1.6_ cg

44. 1.00 m = _100_ cm

45. 4 kg = _4000_ g

46. 729 cm = _7.29_ m

47. 6 g = _600_ cg

48. 56.08 cc = _56.08_ ml

49. 19 g = _.019_ kg

50. 65.3 liters = _65,300_ cc

Passing score is no more than *6* errors. ─○

Chapter 5

Conversions Between Metric and English Units

Section 1   Converting Inches to Centimeters

Many times we must be able to convert English units to metric units and vice versa. For example, many hospitals record a patient's weight in kilograms and his height in centimeters.

Consider the following question:

How many centimeters long is a baby who is 20 inches long?

The conversion unit to use is:

> **1 inch = 2.5 centimeters**

1. If 1 in. equals 2.5 cm, how many centimeters are in 20 in.?

Let's try several problems.

2. Change 95 in. to centimeters.

3. Change 100 in. to centimeters.

4. Change 30 in. to centimeters.

5. Change 36 in. to centimeters.

6. Change 60 in. to centimeters.

7. Change 240 in. to centimeters.

8. Change 1,250 in. to centimeters.

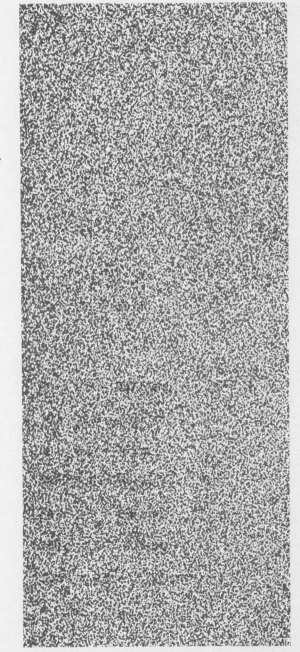

9. Change 300 in. to centimeters.

10. Change 325 in. to centimeters.

Passing score is no more than *1* error.

Section 2   Converting Pounds to Grams

Consider the following question:

How many grams are in a four-pound bag of flour?

The conversion unit to use is:

1 pound = 454 grams

1. If 1 pound equals 454 g, how many grams do 4 pounds equal?

2. Change 10 pounds to grams.

3. Change 88 pounds to grams.

4. Change 32 pounds to grams.

5. Change 100 pounds to grams.

6. Change 1,800 pounds to grams.

7. Change 90 pounds to grams.

8. Change 25 pounds to grams.

9. Change 220 pounds to grams.

10. Change 14 pounds to grams.

Passing score is no more than *1* error.

Section 3   Converting Kilograms to Pounds

Consider the following question:

How many pounds is 4 kilograms?

The conversion unit to use is:

1 kilogram = 2.2 pounds

1. If 1 kg equals 2.2 pounds, how many pounds do 4 kg equal?

2. Change 10 kg to pounds.

3. Change 25 kg to pounds.

4. Change 100 kg to pounds.

5. Change 120 kg to pounds.

6. Change 88 kg to pounds.

7. Change 219 kg to pounds.

8. Change 110 kg to pounds.

9. Change 35 kg to pounds.

10. Change 22 kg to pounds.

Passing score is no more than 1 error.

Section 4 Converting Centimeters to Inches

Consider the following question:

How many inches long is a baby who is 50 centimeters long?

The conversion unit to use is:

1 inch = 2.5 centimeters

1. If 1 in. equals 2.5 cm, how many inches are 50 cm?

2. Change 200 cm to inches.

3. Change 360 cm to inches.

4. Change 1,200 cm to inches.

5. Change 220 cm to inches.

6. Change 900 cm to inches.

7. Change 118 cm to inches.

8. Change 3,000 cm to inches.

9. Change 150 cm to inches.

10. Change 0.75 cm to inches.

Passing score is no more than *1* error.

Section 5 Converting Grams to Pounds

Consider the following question:

How many pounds are in 999 g?

The conversion unit to use is:

1 pound = 454 g

1. If 1 pound equals 454 g, how many pounds are in 999 g?

Whenever you want to convert grams to pounds, divide the number of grams by 454.

Let's try several problems.

2. Change 1,816 g to pounds.

3. Change 9,988 g to pounds.

4. Change 42,676 g to pounds.

5. Change 4,540 g to pounds.

6. Change 39,860 g to pounds.

7. Change 7,718 g to pounds.

8. Change 3,632 g to pounds.

9. Change 908,000 g to pounds.

10. Change 99,880 g to pounds.

Passing score is no more than *1* error.

Section 6 Converting Pounds to Kilograms

Consider the following question:

How many kilograms are in 76 pounds?

The conversion unit to use is:

1 kilogram = 2.2 pounds

1. If 2.2 pounds equals 1 kg, how much does 74.8 pounds equal?

Whenever you want to convert pounds to kilograms, you divide the number of pounds by 2.2.

Let's try several problems.

2. Change 22 pounds to kilograms.

3. Change 55 pounds to kilograms.

4. Change 220 pounds to kilograms.

5. Change 264 pounds to kilograms.

6. Change 48.4 pounds to kilograms.

7. Change 77 pounds to kilograms.

8. Change 242 pounds to kilograms.

9. Change 431.2 pounds to kilograms.

10. Change 176 pounds to kilograms.

Passing score is no more than *1* error.

Section 7   Review

Below are the conversion units needed:

1 in. = 2.5 cm
1 pound = 454 g
1 kg = 2.2 pounds

Now let's try several problems.

1. Change 5,448 g to pounds.

2. Change 66 pounds to kilograms.

3. Change 1,600 in. to centimeters.

4. Change 94 pounds to grams.

5. Change 237.5 cm to inches.

6. Change 200 kg to pounds.

7. Change 29 in. to centimeters.

8. Change 220 pounds to kilograms.

9. Change 0.80 cm to inches.

10. Change 55 pounds to kilograms.

11. How many pounds are in 36 kg?

12. Change 3,632 g to pounds.

13. Change 28 in. to centimeters.

14. Change 242 pounds to kilograms.

15. Change 39,860 g to pounds.

16. Change 6,250 cm to inches.

17. Change 68 kg to pounds.

18. Change 1,800 in. to centimeters.

19. Change 30 kg to pounds.

20. Change 70.4 pounds to kilograms.

Passing score is no more than *4* errors.

Chapter 6

Comparison of the Household and Metric Systems

Although the household system of measurement is not as accurate as the metric system, it is frequently used by the patient at home because he knows what a teaspoonful of medicine is; he knows what drops are; he knows what an ounce is. While he is able to measure these amounts by himself, he might not know how to measure something that was given in metric units. The household system of measurement is an approximate system, because all droppers are not the same size. Likewise, all teaspoons, tablespoons, and glasses are not the same size. However, this system of measurement is quite satisfactory in several instances.

Let us consider how to convert units in the metric system to units in the household system.

The *approximate* conversions are:

Household System		Metric System
20 drops	=	1 ml
1 teaspoonful	=	5 ml
1 tablespoonful	=	15 ml
1 glassful	=	250 ml

1. How many drops are in 1 ml?

2. How many drops are in $\frac{1}{2}$ ml?

3. How many drops are in $\frac{1}{5}$ ml?

4. How many teaspoonfuls are in 30 ml?

5. How many tablespoonfuls are in 30 ml?

6. How many glassfuls are in 500 ml?

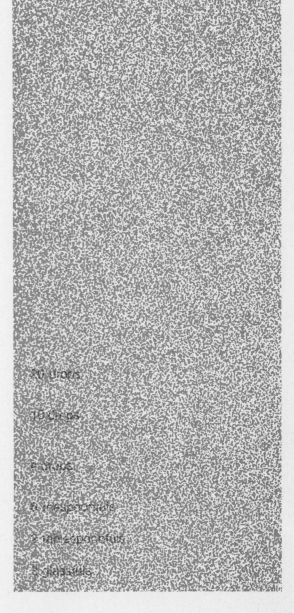

7. How many tablespoonfuls are in 15 ml? |

8. If the doctor prescribed 10 ml, what would you tell the patient to take at home?   2 teaspoonful

9. If the doctor prescribed 15 ml, what would you tell the patient to take at home?   1 tablespoonful

10. If the doctor prescribed 250 ml, what would you tell the patient to take at home?   1 glassful

11. If the doctor prescribed $\frac{1}{10}$ ml, what would you tell the patient to take at home?   10 √15 / 5   2 drops

12. If the doctor prescribed 5 ml, what would you tell the patient to take at home?   1 teaspoonful

13. If the doctor prescribed $\frac{1}{4}$ ml, what would you tell the patient to take at home?   4 √16   4 drops

Passing score is no more than *3* errors.

Chapter 7

Ratio and Proportion

A ratio is simply one number compared to another.

Consider the following instruction:

Please fill this bottle with 1 part water to 2 parts saline solution.

1 part water to 2 parts saline solution represents a ratio of 1 to 2. A ratio of 1 to 2 may be written $1:2$ or $\frac{1}{2}$.

A proportion consists of two ratios that are equal to each other. Read the following:

1 part water to 2 parts saline solution is in the same ratio as 2 parts water to 4 parts saline solution. Since the two ratios are equal, they may be written as a proportion:

$$\frac{1}{2} = \frac{2}{4}$$

Sometimes, one term of a ratio is missing. For instance:

$$\frac{1}{2} = \frac{X}{6}$$

The purpose of this chapter is to teach you how to determine the value of the missing term.

Section 1   How to Determine the Value of *X*

In algebra, *X* represents something that is unknown.

Consider the following problem:

If $2X = 4$,

What does *X* equal?

Here is all you do to solve the problem.

Problem: $2X = 4$; solve for X.

Step 1: $\dfrac{2X}{2} = \dfrac{4}{2}$

Answer: $X = 2$

Read the following carefully:

Problem: $3X = 9$; solve for X.

Step 1: $\dfrac{3X}{3} = \dfrac{9}{3}$

Answer: $X = 3$

In this type of problem, whenever you want to determine the value of X, simply divide both sides of the equation by the number before the X.

Solve for X in each of the following problems.

1. $6X = 48$

2. $4X = 24$

3. $5X = 55$

4. $6X = \dfrac{1}{3}$

5. $7X = 49$

6. $12X = 72$

7. $150 = 10X$

8. $\frac{1}{2}X = \frac{1}{4}$

9. $\frac{1}{2}X = 10$

10. $12X = 144$

11. $15X = 225$

12. $\frac{1}{4}X = 40$

13. $3X = 100$

14. $75 = 3X$

15. $18X = 72$

Passing score is no more than *3* errors.

Section 2 Cross-Multiplying Before Solving for *X*

In algebra, $2X$ represents *2 multiplied by X;* $3X$ represents *3 multiplied by X.*

1. Write 10 multiplied by *X.*

2. Write 12 multiplied by *X.*

3. Write 9 multiplied by *X.*

Consider the following:

$$\frac{X}{4} = \frac{1}{2}$$

Let us consider how to determine the value of *X.*

$$\text{Problem:} \quad \frac{X}{4} = \frac{1}{2}$$

$$\text{Step 1:} \quad 2X = 4 \times 1$$

$$2X = 4$$

$$\text{Step 2:} \quad \frac{2X}{2} = \frac{4}{2}$$

$$\text{Answer:} \quad X = 2$$

Notice that in Step 1, the numerator (X) of the first fraction is multiplied by the denominator (2) of the second fraction, and the denominator of the first fraction (4) is multiplied by the numerator (1) of the second fraction. This is called cross-multiplying.

Consider the following problem:

$$\frac{X}{4} = \frac{12}{24}$$

4. Cross-multiply.

5. Solve for X.

Consider the following:

$$\frac{X}{9} = \frac{4}{6}$$

6. Cross-multiply.

7. Solve for X.

Consider the following:

$$\frac{X}{4} = \frac{5}{2}$$

8. Cross-multiply.

9. Solve for X.

Consider the following:

$$\frac{X}{9} = \frac{4}{18}$$

10. Cross-multiply.

11. Solve for X.

In each of the following problems, cross-multiply and solve for X.

12. $\dfrac{X}{5} = \dfrac{8}{10}$

13. $\dfrac{X}{7} = \dfrac{5}{7}$

14. $\dfrac{3}{X} = \dfrac{9}{6}$

Note: No matter where the X appears, the problem is solved by cross-multiplying.

15. $\dfrac{2}{12} = \dfrac{X}{84}$

16. $\dfrac{9}{X} = \dfrac{3}{9}$

17. $\dfrac{1}{X} = \dfrac{15}{45}$

18. $\dfrac{2}{X} = \dfrac{8}{12}$

19. $\dfrac{1}{4} = \dfrac{X}{44}$

20. $\dfrac{2}{10} = \dfrac{10}{X}$

Passing score is no more than *3* errors.

Consider the following:

$$\dfrac{X}{3\frac{3}{4}} = \dfrac{4}{6}$$

1. Cross-multiply.

2. Solve for *X*.

Notice that we cross-multiply even when there are fractions in the equation.

3. $\dfrac{X}{2\frac{2}{3}} = \dfrac{6}{9}$

4. $\dfrac{X}{\frac{1}{2}} = \dfrac{10}{5}$

5. $\dfrac{\frac{1}{2}}{X} = \dfrac{80}{160}$

6. $\dfrac{\frac{4}{5}}{X} = \dfrac{100}{500}$

7. $\dfrac{X}{15} = \dfrac{1}{2}$

8. $\dfrac{X}{25} = \dfrac{10}{50}$

9. $\dfrac{\frac{2}{3}}{X} = \dfrac{9}{27}$

10. $\dfrac{X}{\frac{1}{3}} = \dfrac{9}{12}$

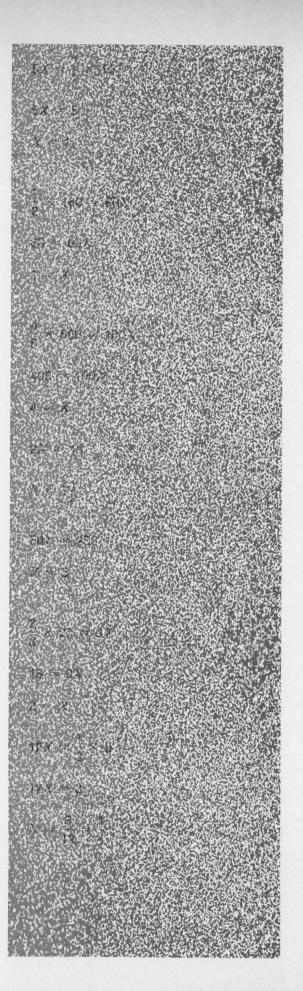

11. $\dfrac{\frac{1}{2}}{10} = \dfrac{X}{20}$

12. $\dfrac{X}{4} = \dfrac{\frac{1}{2}}{40}$

13. $\dfrac{X}{18} = \dfrac{\frac{2}{3}}{6}$

14. $\dfrac{9}{X} = \dfrac{\frac{1}{2}}{36}$

15. $\dfrac{\frac{4}{5}}{10} = \dfrac{X}{20}$

16. Consider the following:

$$\dfrac{\frac{1}{2}}{\frac{1}{10}} = \dfrac{X}{3}$$

Cross-multiply.

17. Now cross-multiply again.

18. Solve for X.

Cross-multiply and solve the following problems.

19. $\dfrac{\frac{1}{3}}{\frac{1}{4}} = \dfrac{X}{4}$

20. $\dfrac{\frac{7}{8}}{\frac{1}{2}} = \dfrac{X}{400}$

21. $\dfrac{\frac{1}{5}}{70} = \dfrac{X}{100}$

22. $\dfrac{\frac{2}{5}}{\frac{1}{2}} = \dfrac{X}{10}$

23. $\dfrac{\frac{1}{3}}{\frac{4}{5}} = \dfrac{X}{90}$

24. $\dfrac{\frac{1}{2}}{\frac{1}{4}} = \dfrac{8}{X}$

25. $\dfrac{\frac{2}{3}}{\frac{1}{5}} = \dfrac{25}{X}$

Passing score is no more than *4* errors.

Chapter 8

Abbreviations Used for Medications

Section 1 Methods of Administering Medications

Medications may be given by one of several different methods, depending on the doctor's order.

Look at the following:

Give 100 mg meperidine IM.

This order may be read as "give 100 milligrams of meperidine intramuscularly."

1. What does the abbreviation IM mean?

Look at the following order:

Give 500 mg aminophylline IV.

This order may be read as "give 500 mg of aminophylline intravenously."

2. What does the abbreviation IV mean?

Look at the following order:

Give 45 U insulin subq.

This order may be read as "give 45 units of insulin subcutaneously."

3. What does the abbreviation subq indicate?

Look at the following order:

Give Librium 10 mg.

This order may be read as "give 10 mg of Librium orally."

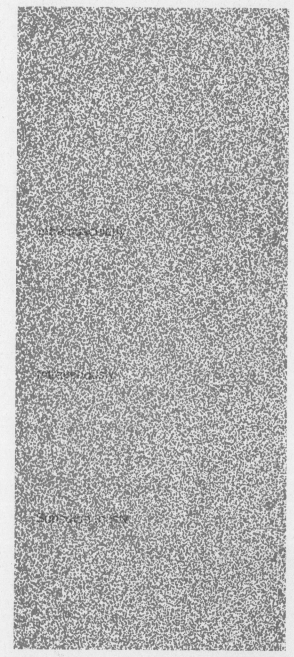

4. If no method of administration is indicated, how should the medication be administered?

5. How should the following medication be administered?

> Give 15 cc of Gelusil orally.

Note that for oral medications, the word orally may or may not be indicated.

What does each of the following abbreviations indicate?

6. IV

7. Subq

8. IM

What abbreviations should be used for the following methods of administration?

9. Subcutaneously

10. Orally

11. Intravenously

12. Intramuscularly

Passing score is *0* errors.

Section 2 Frequency of Administering Medications

The frequency of administration of medications is indicated by abbreviations included in the medication order. The medication may be ordered once a day, twice a day, before meals, after meals, at bedtime, or even immediately.

Look at the following medication order:

> Give 75 mg Demerol IM p.r.n.

The order may be read as "give 75 milligrams of Demerol intramuscularly when necessary."

1. What does the abbreviation p.r.n. indicate?

2. What does the abbreviation IM indicate?

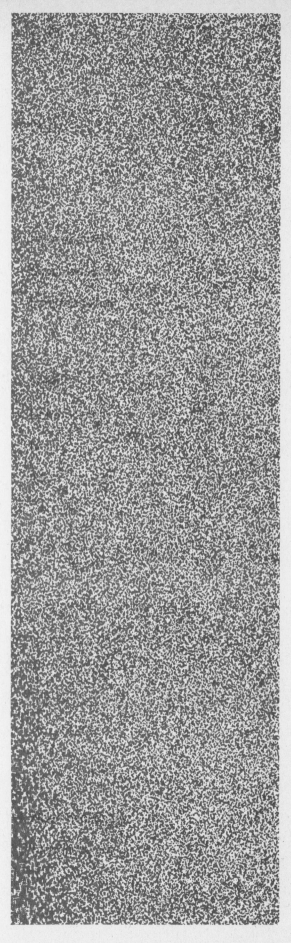

Look at the following medication order:

Give stilbestrol 0.5 mg t.i.d.

This order may be read as "give 0.5 milligram of stilbestrol orally three times a day."

3. What does the abbreviation t.i.d. indicate?

4. How do you know that the medication is to be given orally?

Look at the following order:

Give Orinase 0.5 g b.i.d.

This order may be read as "give 0.5 gram of Orinase orally twice a day."

5. What does the abbreviation b.i.d. indicate?

6. What does the abbreviation t.i.d. indicate?

Look at the following order:

Give tetracycline 250 mg q.i.d.

This order may be read as "give 250 milligrams of tetracycline orally four times a day."

7. What does the abbreviation q.i.d. indicate?

8. How may "three times a day" be abbreviated?

9. How may "twice a day" be abbreviated?

10. How may "four times a day" be abbreviated?

Look at the following order:

Give 15 cc Amphojel q.h.

This order may be read as "give 15 cc of Amphojel orally every hour."

11. What does the abbreviation q.h. indicate?

Look at the following order:

Give 15 cc aluminum hydroxide gel q.2h.

This order may be read as "give 15 cc of aluminum hydroxide gel orally every two hours."

12. What does the abbreviation q.2h. indicate?

13. What is the abbreviation for "every hour"?

14. What is the abbreviation for "every two hours"?

15. What would you expect to be the abbreviation for "every three hours"?

Look at the following order:

Give Gantrisin 0.5 g a.c.

This order may be read as "give one-half gram of Gantrisin orally before meals."

16. What does the abbreviation a.c. indicate?

Look at the following order:

Give ascorbic acid 250 mg p.c.

This order may be read as "give 250 milligrams of ascorbic acid orally after meals."

17. What does the abbreviation p.c. indicate?

18. What does the abbreviation a.c. indicate?

Look at the following order:

Give insulin 40 U IM q.a.m.

This order may be read as "give forty units of insulin intramuscularly every morning."

19. What does the abbreviation q.a.m. indicate?

Look at the following order:

Give Diuril 500 mg q.d.

This order may be read as "give five hundred milligrams of Diuril orally every day."

20. What does the abbreviation q.d. indicate?

Look at the following order:

Give 100 mg Tuinal h.s.

This order may be read as "give 100 mg of Tuinal orally at bedtime."

21. What does the abbreviation h.s. indicate?

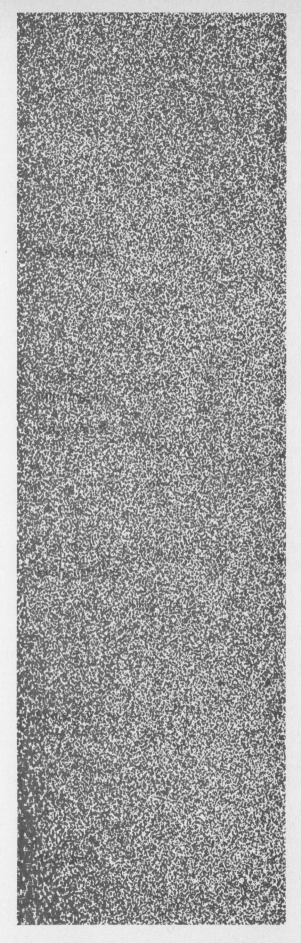

Look at the following order:

Give Demerol 50 mg IM stat.

This order may be read as "give fifty milligrams of Demerol intramuscularly immediately."

22. What does the abbreviation stat. indicate?

Now let us go over these abbreviations. Indicate the meaning of each of the following abbreviations.*

1. p.c.

2. b.i.d.

3. q.3h.

4. stat.

5. h.s.

6. a.c.

7. t.i.d.

8. q.h.

9. q.i.d.

10. p.r.n.

11. q.a.m.

12. q.d.

13. q.2h.

For each of the following orders, indicate the method of administration and also the frequency of administration.

1. Give 600,000 U procaine penicillin IM, b.i.d.

2. Give 30 U N.P.H. insulin subq., q.a.m.

3. Give 0.1 mg digitoxin, q.a.m.

4. Give 300 mg ferrous sulfate, oral, t.i.d., p.c.

5. Give 15 cc Maalox q.h.

6. Give 0.6 mg scopolamine subq, stat.

* On computer printouts these abbreviations are usually capitalized, and without periods between letters. Thus, p.c. is abbreviated as PC; b.i.d., as BID; and q.3h., as Q3H.

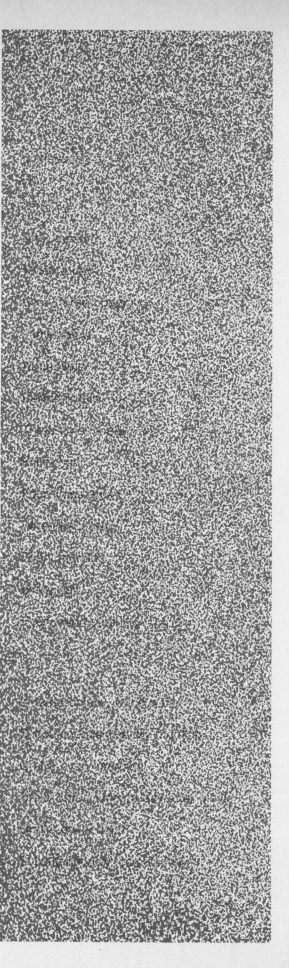

7. Give 250 mg tetracycline orally q.i.d.

8. Give 100 mg Tuinal h.s.

9. Give 30 mg Talwin IM, p.r.n.

10. Give 25 mg Aldactone t.i.d.

11. Give 0.5 g Gantrisin orally a.c.

12. Give 8 cc Phenergan expectorant q.3h.

13. Give 40 U insulin subq., q.a.m.

14. Give 50 mg Demerol IM, stat.

15. Give 250 mg Chloromycetin t.i.d.

16. Give 5 mg dextroamphetamine sulfate, oral, a.c.

17. Give 10 mg Librium q.i.d.

18. Give 0.5 g Diuril q.a.m.

19. Give 10 mg morphine sulfate IM, p.r.n.

20. Give 0.25 mg digoxin q.d.

21. Give 200 mg quinidine sulfate orally, q.2h.

22. Give 10 cc Benylin expectorant q.3h.

23. Give 0.5 g Orinase b.i.d.

24. Give 100 mg secobarbital h.s.

25. Give 500 mg aminophylline IV, stat.

26. Give 250 mg ascorbic acid oral, p.c.

27. Give 75 mg Demerol IM, p.r.n.

28. Give 0.1 mg digitoxin q.a.m.

29. Give 100 mg thiamine hydrochloride IM, q.d.

30. Give 15 cc Gelusil q.h.

Passing score is no more than *2* errors.

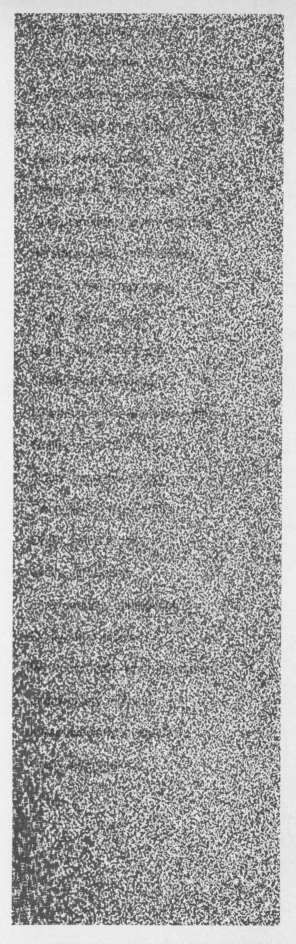

Section 3 The 24-Hour Clock

Many institutions are using the 24-hour clock because it's a better way of clearly specifying when to give medications.

For example, with the 24-hour clock, 8 A.M. is 0800, 8:30 A.M. is 0830, and 9:15 A.M. is 0915.

P.M. time is 1200 plus the hour and minutes. For instance, 1 P.M. is 1300, 2:30 P.M. is 1430, and 9:45 P.M. is 2145.

Change the following to 24-hour times.

1. 2 A.M.   0200

2. 9 P.M.   2100

3. 4 P.M.   1600

4. 7 A.M.   0700

5. 9:30 A.M. 0930

6. 7:30 P.M. 1930

Change the following from 24-hour times to common times.

7. 0800   8:00am

8. 1700   5:00 pm

9. 0730   7:30am

10. 2300   11:00 pm

11. 2030   8:30 pm

12. 1000   10:00am

Chapter 9

Some Medical/Nursing Applications of Computers

The chances are excellent that your hospital's pharmacy is already using or is going to be using an automated data processing system for filling medication orders. As a result, you need to know certain fundamental things about computers and how they work.

Let's begin with a task that might seem quite simple. Assume that a computer in the pharmacy prints medication labels. For example, look at Figure 9-1 (page 94).

Refer to Figure 9-1 as you try to answer the next series of questions.

1. The name of what medication appears on the four labels?

2. According to the schedule, how frequently is the medication to be administered?

3. When was the medication first to be given?

4. When was the medication prepared?

5. Who prepared the medication?

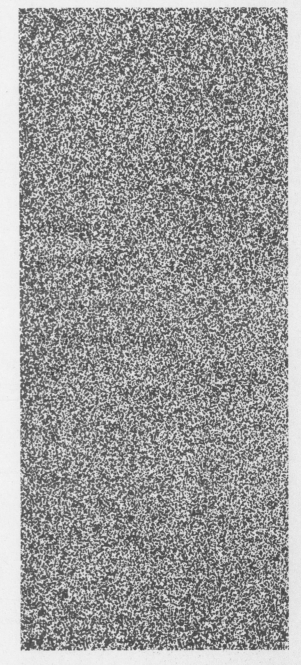

```
HAGBERG    ELOIZABETH                    E451  B

AMPICILLIN  1  G  IV  MINNI  BOTTLE

SCHED  Q6H                      2100  10/21/82
PREPARED  AT:  1400  10/21/82  BY:  JWB
     - - - EXPIRES  AFTER  36  HOURS - - -
               REFRIGERATE
```

```
HAGBERG    ELOIZABETH                    E451  B

AMPICILLIN  1  G  IV  MINNI  BOTTLE

SCHED  Q6H                      0300  10/22/82
PREPARED  AT:  1400  10/21/82  BY:  JWB
     - - - EXPIRES  AFTER  36  HOURS - - -
               REFRIGERATE
```

```
HAGBERG    ELOIZABETH                    E451  B

AMPICILLIN  1  G  IV  MINNI  BOTTLE

SCHED  Q6H                      0900  10/22/82
PREPARED  AT:  1400  10/21/82  BY:  JWB
     - - - EXPIRES  AFTER  36  HOURS - - -
               REFRIGERATE
```

```
HAGBERG    ELOIZABETH                    E451  B

AMPICILLIN  1  G  IV  MINNI  BOTTLE

SCHED  Q6H                      1500  10/22/82
PREPARED  AT:  1400  10/21/82  BY:  JWB
     - - - EXPIRES  AFTER  36  HOURS - - -
               REFRIGERATE
```

Figure 9-1. (*Courtesy of Greenwich Hospital, Greenwich, Conn.*)

6. How long is the medication good?

7. The IV bottles will be sent to the floor. What should the nurse do with the medication?

As you can see, this seemingly simply label contains considerable information.

8. How many labels did the computer prepare for a single medication order?

Notice that the computer produced a label for each bottle that was prepared at 1400 on 10/21/82.

These four labels illustrate one of the significant advantages of using a computer. In the above example, the medication order is for four IV bottles. The pharmacy needs a label for each bottle. If someone typed the four labels on a typewriter, the person would type almost the same information four times. By way of illustration, try to answer the next questions.

9. Does the name change from label to label?

10. Does the room change?

11. Does the medication change?

12. What is the only information that does change?

One of the things to keep in mind about using a computer is that it eliminates the need to type the same information again and again. With a computer, you only type the information once. From then on, the computer is able to print the information whenever it's needed. For instance, assume the operator keys in the name, room, and bed for the first label. The computer can then use the same information on the 2nd, 3rd, and 4th labels. *The elimination of the need to repeatedly type the same information is one of the advantages of using a computer.*

Let's consider another advantage. *Look again at Figure 9-1 and carefully read the name, room, and bed on the first label.*

Using an ordinary typewriter, a person could easily make a mistake on any of the four labels. With a computer, you can be sure that the same information will appear on every label. *Look at the way Elizabeth has been spelled on the four labels.*

Notice that Elizabeth is misspelled. As you can see, the same misspelling occurs on all of the labels. This illustrates an important point about computers. If the person who originally enters the data into the computer does not catch a mistake, the error will appear whenever the data is printed. *Being consistent* is another of the computer's advantages. Keep in

mind that if the data is entered correctly, you can be sure it will be correct whenever it's printed. On the other hand, that's not true when a human being uses a typewriter. For example, a person could spell the name correctly on the first label and misspell it on the second.

Incidentally, a well-designed computer system anticipates human errors and provides an easy way to make corrections. For example, there is usually a special program for each file, which is sometimes called a *maintenance program*. If the nurse on the floor discovers that a patient's name is misspelled, the spelling can be changed quite easily using the maintenance program.

Thus far, you've learned two advantages of using a computer. To make sure you know them, try to answer the next questions.

13. What's the first advantage you have learned?

14. What's the second advantage?

Let's consider how information is entered into the computer. Look at Figure 9-2.

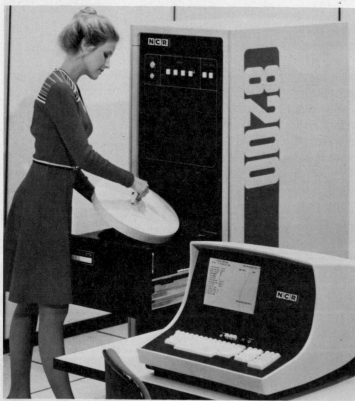

Figure 9-2. Information is entered into the computer by typing it on the terminal's keyboard. The information being entered will also appear on the screen. (*Courtesy of NCR Corporation, Dayton, Ohio.*)

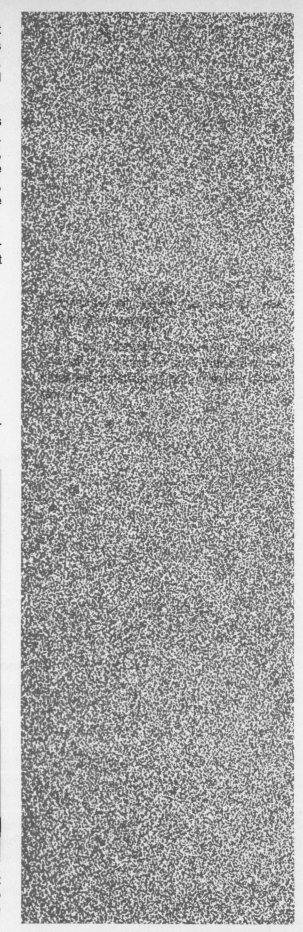

```
PATIENT NUMBER:
MEDICATION:
SCHEDULE:
STARTING TIME:
STARTING DATE:
EXPIRES:
HOW TO STORE:
```

Figure 9-3.

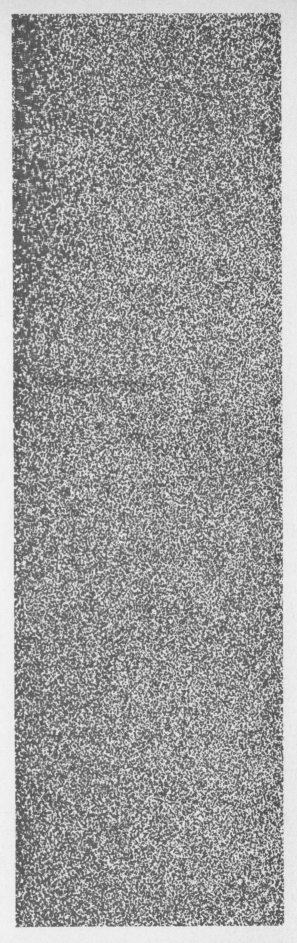

A terminal is connected to the computer. A terminal is frequently called a CRT, which stands for Cathode Ray Tube. Let's trace what happens from the time the pharmacy receives a medication order to the printing of the label on the computer. Look at Figure 9-3.

15. According to the prompts shown on the CRT, what is the first thing the operator needs to enter?

The patient number illustrates another important computer concept. Consider the following problem. Suppose the operator enters the wrong patient number. For example, the operator enters the number of a patient who's been discharged. Here's another possibility. The operator mistakenly enters the number for John Jones instead of for Mary Smith. You certainly wouldn't want the medication for John Jones going to Mary Smith.

Please read the following information carefully.

A record is stored on the computer's file for every patient in the hospital. When the operator enters a patient number, the computer checks the file to make sure the patient is actually occupying a bed. If the patient is not occupying a bed, the computer displays a message on the CRT to let the operator know there's been a mistake.

The second possible mistake involves the operator entering the number of a different patient. For example, the operator should enter the number for Mary Smith and mistakenly enters the number for John Jones. The computer has no way of catching this kind of mistake. However, a well-designed computer system assumes that operators are going to make mistakes. Therefore, certain safeguards are built into the system to enable the operator to catch mistakes. For example, as you look at Figure 9-4, assume that the operator entered a patient number. *Then, notice that the computer displays the patient's name on the CRT.* By comparing the name on the CRT to the name on the medication order, the operator will be able to catch the mistake.

```
PATIENT NUMBER:    12345
                   JOHN  JONES
```

Figure 9-4.

In the example in Figure 9-4, the operator was supposed to enter patient number 54321 (Mary Smith). By mistake, the operator entered 12345 (John Jones). Both patients have been admitted to the hospital. As you can see, after finding the record for Patient 12345 the computer displayed the patient's name on the CRT so that the operator could verify the patient's name.

Displaying the name makes it easy for the operator to catch the error. This example illustrates another important advantage of using a computer. Try to answer the next question.

16. What advantage do you think is illustrated in the above example?

As you look at Figure 9-5, notice the information that is printed on the first line of the label.

```
HAGBERG    ELOIZABETH                 E451  B

AMPICILLIN  1  G  IV  MINNI  BOTTLE

SCHED  Q6H                   2100  10/21/82
PREPARED  AT:  1400  10/21/82  BY:  JWB
     - - - EXPIRES  AFTER  36  HOURS - - -
                 REFRIGERATE
```

Figure 9-5. (*Courtesy of Greenwich Hospital, Greenwich, Conn.*)

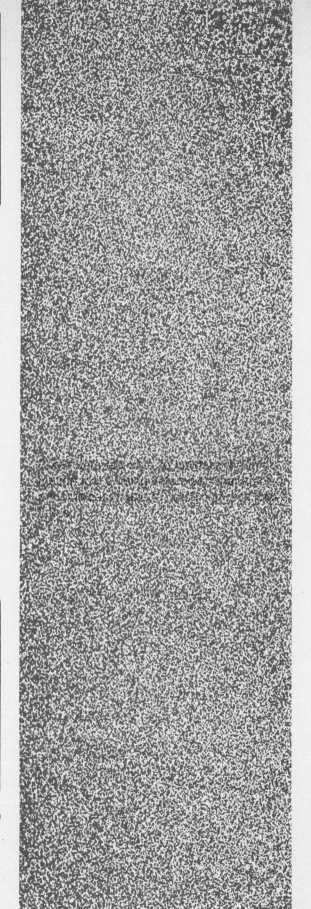

Notice that the computer is going to print the last name, first name, room, and bed on the first line. However, the operator *only has to enter the patient number.* With just the patient number, the computer is able to print the first line of the label. Let's consider why that's possible. Look at Figure 9-6.

```
PATIENT NUMBER:    54321
LAST NAME:         HAGBERG
FIRST NAME:        ELOIZABETH
ROOM:              E451
BED:               B
```

Figure 9-6. The computer stores a record for each patient with the above information. (For training purposes only.)

The computer is able to print the name, room, and bed on the first line of the label because the information is already on file. This illustrates another feature of using the computer. Try to answer the next question.

17. What advantage is illustrated in the above example?

Let's consider another important computer concept. Look at Figure 9-7.

```
HAGBERG   ELOIZABETH                E451 B

AMPICILLIN 1 G IV MINNI BOTTLE

SCHED Q6H                    2100 10/21/82
PREPARED AT: 1400 10/21/82 BY: JWB
    ---EXPIRES AFTER 36 HOURS---
              REFRIGERATE
```

Figure 9-7. (*Courtesy of Greenwich Hospital, Greenwich, Conn.*)

18. According to the label, how much ampicillin is to be administered in each IV bottle?

One of the things the computer can do is to make sure that the dosage is within an acceptable range. Let's consider how a computer recognizes whether a dosage is within an acceptable range. Look at Figure 9-8.

```
MEDICATION:
MINIMUM DOSAGE:
MAXIMUM DOSAGE:
```

Figure 9-8. The computer stores a record for each medication with the above information. (For training purposes only.)

Assume that the computer is storing certain information about every medication stocked in the pharmacy. As you can see, the record indicates the minimum and maximum dosages. When the operator enters an order for a particular medication, the computer goes to the record for that medication. If the dosage that the operator enters is less than the minimum the computer has on file, or greater than the maximum, the computer recognizes that the order is not within the acceptable range.

The record shown in Figure 9-8 is a simple example. Let's consider what's involved in a slightly more sophisticated system. Suppose that the acceptable dosage for a particular medication depends upon the weight and age of the patient. Think carefully as you try to answer the next questions.

19. Assuming that the appropriate dosage depends upon the patient's age and weight, what would the computer need to know about the patient in order to determine whether the operator had entered an acceptable dosage?

20. Where do you think the computer might store the patient's age and weight?

Think carefully as you try to answer the next question.

21. Assume the computer is storing the age and weight of each patient. What information about each medication must the computer store in order to determine whether a particular dosage is appropriate for a particular patient?

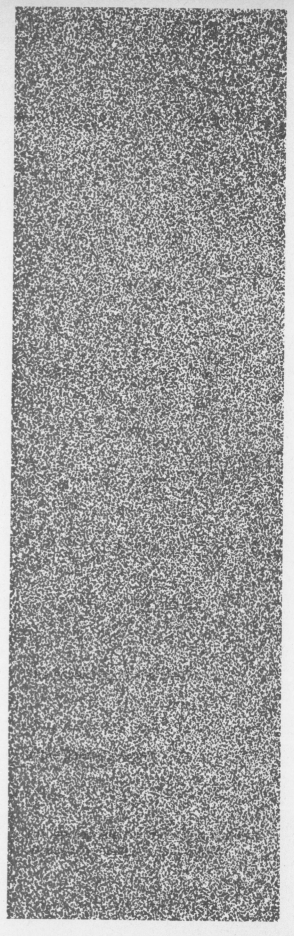

In other words, the computer must actually store a table of the appropriate dosages for each age and weight.

As you can see from this illustration, computer systems can easily become quite complex. Let's consider one additional factor. Suppose the appropriate dosage also depends upon the patient's allergies and any other medication the patient is receiving. In highly sophisticated hospital systems, the computer actually checks the medication order to make sure that it's appropriate to combine the new medication with other medications the patient is already receiving.

Look at the third line of each label in Fig. 9-9 (page 102).

Notice the schedule and time on the four labels. These labels illustrate another advantage of using a computer. If a person had to type these labels, the typist would have to spend a certain amount of time calculating when the medication should be given for each label. Using a computer, the machine automatically calculates when to give the medication based upon the starting time and the schedule.

The Greenwich Hospital in Stamford, Conn., is one of the hospitals using a small computer in its pharmacy to produce medication labels. Of course, it takes considerable funds to develop a complex computer system for a hospital. As a matter of fact, a hospital could never justify the cost of a computer system based upon the computer's ability to eliminate the need to type labels. The real savings occur in the powerful reports the computer can generate from the information that a pharmacist enters for every medication order. For example, scan the information on Figure 9-10.

Every medication order the operator enters into the computer is stored in a computer file. The report in Figure 9-10 illustrates another important feature of using a computer. Think carefully before you try to answer the next question.

```
    HAGBERG    ELOIZABETH                    E451 B

    AMPICILLIN 1 G IV MINNI BOTTLE

    SCHED Q6H                          2100  10/21/82
    PREPARED AT: 1400  10/21/82  BY: JWB
        - - - EXPIRES AFTER 36 HOURS - - -
                      REFRIGERATE
```

```
    HAGBERG    ELOIZABETH                    E451 B

    AMPICILLIN 1 G IV MINNI BOTTLE

    SCHED Q6H                          0300  10/22/82
    PREPARED AT: 1400  10/21/82  BY: JWB
        - - - EXPIRES AFTER 36 HOURS - - -
                      REFRIGERATE
```

```
    HAGBERG    ELOIZABETH                    E451 B

    AMPICILLIN 1 G IV MINNI BOTTLE

    SCHED Q6H                          0900  10/22/82
    PREPARED AT: 1400  10/21/82  BY: JWB
        - - - EXPIRES AFTER 36 HOURS - - -
                      REFRIGERATE
```

```
    HAGBERG    ELOIZABETH                    E451 B

    AMPICILLIN 1 G IV MINNI BOTTLE

    SCHED Q6H                          1500  10/22/82
    PREPARED AT: 1400  10/21/82  BY: JWB
        - - - EXPIRES AFTER 36 HOURS - - -
                      REFRIGERATE
```

Figure 9-9. (*Courtesy of Greenwich Hospital, Greenwich, Conn.*)

```
   81123341                          PHARMACY PROFILE              10/14/82  1529   PAGE 01
GARTH   ALTHEA L.   AGE 52   ADM-10/14/82   MCCALLEY, S                     ROOM-BED-W513 A
   ALLERGIES:

                                                   STARTING        ENDING
     MEDICATION              DOSE   IV IN RT SCHED  TIME    DATE    TIME    DATE   COUNT   REC
*FOLIC ACID 1 MG TABLETS UD   1 TAB    01 PO Q DAY  0900   101482  0000   000000    2 3197
*THIAMINE 100 MG TABLET UD    1 TAB    01 PO Q DAY  0900   101482  0000   000000    2 1136
*Z-BEC TABLET UD              1 TAB    01 PO Q DAY  0900   101482  0000   000000    2 0991
*THYROID 120 MG TABLET UD     1 TAB    01 PO Q DAY  0900   101482  0000   000000    2 1101


*TRIAMINIC DM LIQUID         5 ML Q4H  01 PO        0900   101482  0000   000000    1 0389
                                            BEDSIDE
*TESSALON PERLES 100 MG      100 MG TID 01 PO PRN   0000   101482  0000   000000    0 4277
```

Figure 9-10. (*Courtesy of Greenwich Hospital, Greenwich, Conn.*)

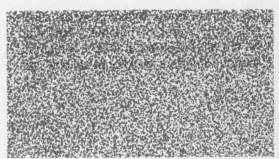

22. What important advantage of using a computer is illustrated by the report shown in Figure 9-10.

Actually, at the Greenwich Hospital, the computer is able to produce many important reports using the same information again and again. For example, look at Figure 9-11.

```
                          DISCHARGE SUMMARY

   81106924                    WHYTE   ROBERT                          2/15/83

                                                            NO.
           DRUG DESCRIPTION             DOSE      RT   COST  USED   EXT.
DEXAMETHASONE 0.5 MG TABLET UD         1 TAB      PO   0.25   25     6.25
DEXAMETHASONE 1.5 MG TABLET UD         1 TAB      PO   0.25   25     6.25
PLATINOL DRUG PROTOCOL                               150.00    1   150.00
MUTAMYCIN INJ 5 MG                     10 MG         148.90    1   148.90
IV SODIUM CHLORIDE .9% 250 ML          VP-16 70 MG    8.50    1     8.50
IV CATHETER                                           2.50    7    17.50
MYCOSTATIN SUSP 100,000 U/ML (60 ML)   5 CC       PO   5.00    5    25.00
HEPARIN LOCK 100 UNITS/VIAL            2              5.00    1     5.00
VISTARIL 25 MG CAPSULE UD              1 CAP      PO   0.40   82    32.80
FLEET ENEMA-ADULT                                PR   1.00    1     1.00
PREDNISONE 5 MG TAB UD (DELTASONE)     2 TAB      PO   0.50   31    15.50
NON FORMULARY DRUG                     HEXAMETHYL     0.00    1     0.00
IRRIGATE NORMAL SALINE 1000 ML         1             4.00    2     8.00
PRO-BANTHINE 15 MG TABLET UD           1 TAB      PO   0.25   62    15.50
IV CATHETER                                           2.50    2     5.00
IV SODIUM CHLORIDE .9% 500 ML                         8.50    1     8.50
METAMUCIL POWDER 14 OZ                 15 GM QD   PO  11.75    1    11.75
VISTARIL 25 MG CAPSULE UD              25 MG QID  PO   0.40    6     2.40
LANOXIN 0.25 MG TABLET UD              2 TAB      PO   0.50   29    14.50
LANOXIN 0.25 MG TABLET UD              1 TAB      PO   0.25    5     1.25

                                                     TOTAL   483.60
```

Figure 9-11. (*Courtesy of Greenwich Hospital, Greenwich, Conn.*)

```
----FILL LIST----                                              11:17
PATIENT NAME    ROOM-BED
              MEDICATION          QTY      SCHEDULE     DOSE      ROUTE

KOELLMER    JOHN    E437 A

    CATAPRES 0.1 MG TABLET          4       BIDAC      2 TAB      PO
    LANOXIN 0.125 MG TABLET UD      1       Q DAY      1
    K-LYTE/CL 25 MEQ EFFERVES TABLET 1      Q DAY      1
    LASIX 40 MG TABLET UD           1       Q DAY      1
    PERSANTINE 25 MG TABLET UD      6       TID        2 TAB      PO
    PREDNISONE 20 MG TABLET UD      2       Q DAY      2          PO
    AMPICILLIN 250 MG CAPSULE UD    8       QID        2
```

Figure 9-12. (*Courtesy of Greenwich Hospital, Greenwich, Conn.*)

One report that is especially important to the nurses on the floor is shown in Figure 9-12. Scan the report carefully.

Nurses on the floor use this report to make sure that the patients receive the appropriate medication at the right time.

The Drug Ordering System at the Rockland Psychiatric Center

The Rockland Psychiatric Center is located about 25 miles from New York City. It's a mental institution with 1,600 beds. There are approximately 1,400 long-term patients, 500 new patients a year, and more than 100 doctors on the staff. Making sure that a patient receives the appropriate medication is complicated because more than one physician may be taking care of the same patient. For example, please scan Figure 9-13.

1. How many doctors prescribed medication for Thomas Jefferson?

Looking at the drug therapy program from the patient's point of view, there are important questions to ask when more than one medication is being administered to the same patient.

2. What is one of the questions that needs to be asked when two medications are prescribed for the same patient?

3. What's another question that needs to be asked?

At the Institute, a special committee determines the recommended maximum dosage for each medication. Generally speaking, doctors should order dosages within the recommended range.

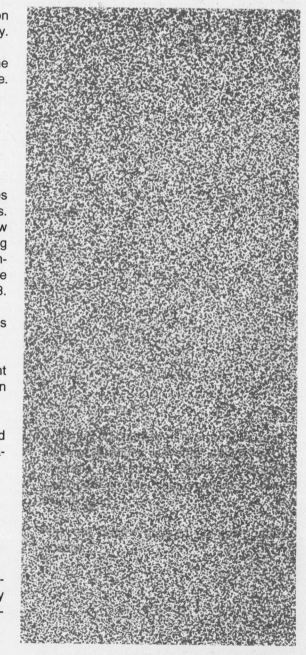

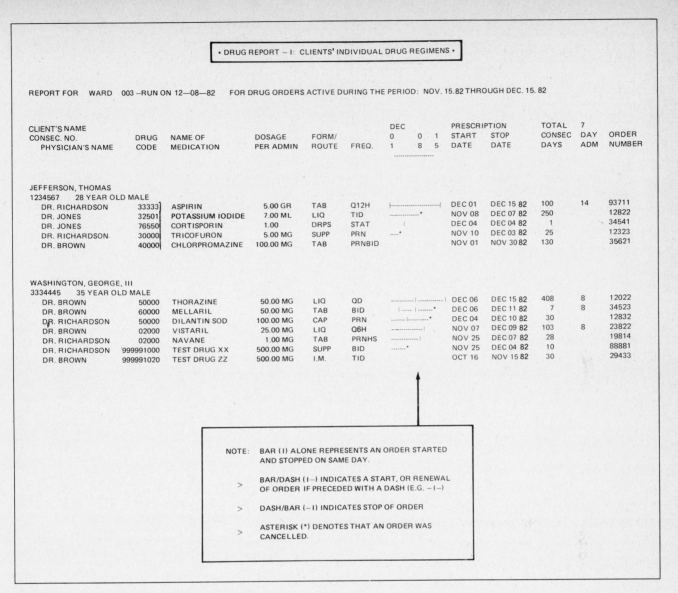

REPORT FOR   WARD   003 —RUN ON 12—08—82   FOR DRUG ORDERS ACTIVE DURING THE PERIOD: NOV. 15.82 THROUGH DEC. 15. 82

CLIENT'S NAME CONSEC. NO. PHYSICIAN'S NAME	DRUG CODE	NAME OF MEDICATION	DOSAGE PER ADMIN	FORM/ ROUTE	FREQ.	DEC 01 18 15	PRESCRIPTION START DATE	STOP DATE	TOTAL CONSEC DAYS	7 DAY ADM	ORDER NUMBER
JEFFERSON, THOMAS 1234567 28 YEAR OLD MALE											
DR. RICHARDSON	33333	ASPIRIN	5.00 GR	TAB	Q12H	|------------------|	DEC 01	DEC 15 82	100	14	93711
DR. JONES	32501	POTASSIUM IODIDE	7.00 ML	LIQ	TID	------------*	NOV 08	DEC 07 82	250		12822
DR. JONES	76550	CORTISPORIN	1.00	DRPS	STAT	|	DEC 04	DEC 04 82	1		34541
DR. RICHARDSON	30000	TRICOFURON	5.00 MG	SUPP	PRN	----*	NOV 10	DEC 03 82	25		12323
DR. BROWN	40000	CHLORPROMAZINE	100.00 MG	TAB	PRNBID		NOV 01	NOV 30 82	130		35621
WASHINGTON, GEORGE, III 3334445 35 YEAR OLD MALE											
DR. BROWN	50000	THORAZINE	50.00 MG	LIQ	QD	----------|---------- |	DEC 06	DEC 15 82	408	8	12022
DR. BROWN	60000	MELLARIL	50.00 MG	TAB	BID	|------ |-------*	DEC 06	DEC 11 82	7	8	34523
DR. RICHARDSON	50000	DILANTIN SOD	100.00 MG	CAP	PRN	------|--------*	DEC 04	DEC 10 82	30		12832
DR. BROWN	02000	VISTARIL	25.00 MG	LIQ	Q6H	---------------|	NOV 07	DEC 09 82	103	8	23822
DR. RICHARDSON	02000	NAVANE	1.00 MG	TAB	PRNHS	-------------|	NOV 25	DEC 07 82	28		19814
DR. RICHARDSON	999991000	TEST DRUG XX	500.00 MG	SUPP	BID	-------*	NOV 25	DEC 04 82	10		88881
DR. BROWN	999991020	TEST DRUG ZZ	500.00 MG	I.M.	TID		OCT 16	NOV 15 82	30		29433

NOTE: BAR (I) ALONE REPRESENTS AN ORDER STARTED AND STOPPED ON SAME DAY.

> BAR/DASH (I–) INDICATES A START, OR RENEWAL OF ORDER IF PRECEDED WITH A DASH (E.G. –I–)

> DASH/BAR (–I) INDICATES STOP OF ORDER

> ASTERISK (*) DENOTES THAT AN ORDER WAS CANCELLED.

Figure 9-13. (*Courtesy of Rockland Research Institute, Orangeburg, N.Y.*)

4. What's another question to ask about a medication order?

The special committee also determines the recommended minimum and maximum time periods for administering each drug.

As you can imagine, using pencil and paper to keep track of the drug orders for 1,600 patients would be an overwhelming and expensive clerical task. However, it is easy and economical for a computer. In simple terms, here is the way the computerized drug-ordering system works at the Rockland Psychiatric Center.

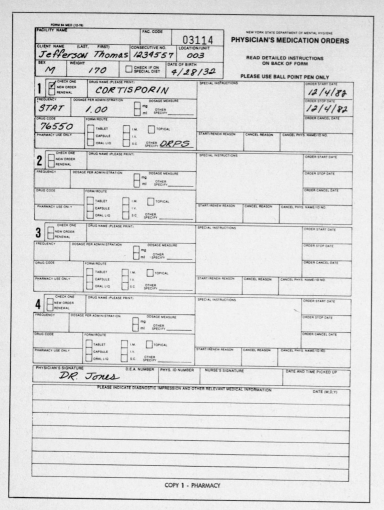

Figure 9-14. (*Courtesy of Rockland Research Institute, Orangeburg, N.Y.*)

The physician orders medication using the form shown in Figure 9-14. Before continuing, please scan the information that the doctor enters on the order.

Assume that the information that the doctor enters on the form is fed into the computer. (You will learn how data gets into the computer shortly.)

When the computer receives a medication order for a patient, it goes to the patient's drug file, which is stored on the computer. (You will learn how the computer stores the patient's drug record shortly.)

Please read the following carefully.

The hospital's committee establishes certain rules for each medication. For instance, Haldol and lithium carbonate should not be given to the same patient. Similarly, the committee establishes the range of dosage and the duration. *The rules that the committee establishes are stored in the computer.*

When a drug order for a particular patient is fed into the computer, the machine checks to make sure that the medication does not violate any of the rules. For example, when the computer receives an order for an antianxiety drug, it will check the drug file to determine if the patient is already receiving an antianxiety drug.

Whenever the computer finds a medication order that violates the hospital's rules, the computer prints a message on a report that is sent to the doctor who ordered the medication.

The advantages of using a computer for this kind of checking are obvious. For a human being in the pharmacy to check each drug order against the patient's drug record would be a time-consuming task in a 6,500-bed hospital. However, when the patient's drug records are on the computer, it takes the machine *less than a second* to check the new drug order against the medication the patient is already receiving.

Let us consider a second important aspect of this computer application. At Rockland State Hospital, there is continuous research to determine which drugs are most effective for specific mental problems. In addition, studies are proceeding to determine whether certain drugs cause adverse reactions when combined with other drugs.

For the moment, assume that the research experts have just discovered that Drug A causes an adverse reaction when combined with Drug B for patients who have diabetes. As soon as the finding has been established, the information will be published in a medical bulletin to alert the doctors on the staff. However, doctors are busy taking care of patients. Because their time is limited, they may not read the bulletin immediately. Here is an example of how the computer can be enormously helpful.

As you may recall, in the Rockland State Hospital, whenever the doctor writes an order, the computer checks the patient's records to determine what medication the patient is already receiving. The computer also checks the new medication to make sure it does not violate any of the rules that the committee has established. *When the research experts establish that Drug A should not be combined with Drug B for patients who have diabetes, this rule is fed into the computer.*

From the instant the new rule has been put into the computer, *the computer will check each order for Drug A to make sure it is not being combined with Drug B for a patient who has diabetes.* Whenever the computer finds a violation of the rule, it prints a message on a report to notify the doctor.

Here is the important point. Without the computer, how quickly a patient benefits from the latest research depends on when the doctor reads the medical bulletin. With the computer, every patient in the hospital benefits immediately from the research. Here is the reason. Once the new rule is put into the computer, the doctor will be alerted whenever an order violates the rule. As you can see, the computer provides an immediate improvement in patient care and makes it easier for the doctor.

Entering Data Into the Computer

Now let us consider the computer itself. Information can be fed into the computer in a number of ways. For example, data can be punched into cards. However, feeding information into the computer from punched cards can create certain problems. For example, errors may be punched into the cards.

The prescription is supposed to be for PATIENT 1111. However, the keypunch operator punches 2222 for the PATIENT IDENTIFICATION.

Letters can be punched in amount fields. For example, instead of key punching 5.00 into the card, the operator punches 5.AA.

Because errors are likely to occur, people who design computer systems write special routines to cause the computer to check the validity of the information that is read from the punched cards. Whenever the computer finds an error, it rejects the card and prints an error message on a VALIDATION REPORT. For example,

If the computer found 5.AA for an AMOUNT, it would reject the card and print a message.

However, analyzing errors from the messages printed on a report and making the appropriate corrections takes time and can be quite cumbersome. Think of what is involved. Someone has to go through the report and determine what correction should be made; the correction must be punched into a new card, fed into the computer, and revalidated. To further complicate matters, there can be new errors in the correction card.

As the cost of computer equipment has gone down, newer ways have been developed to make it easier to get information into the computer.

Notice that Figure 9-15 shows a nurse sitting at a terminal. This type of terminal is known as a CRT. (CRT stands for Cathode Ray Tube.) The CRT terminal is connected to a computer.

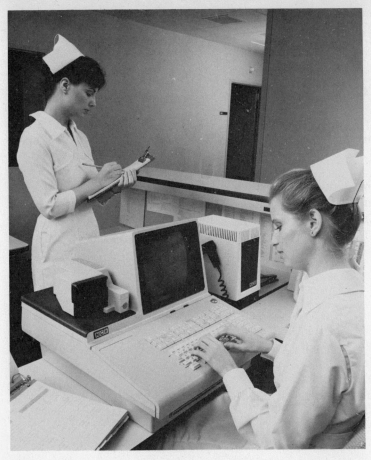

Figure 9-15. Use of a CRT terminal. (*Courtesy of NCR Corporation, Dayton, Ohio.*)

One of the advantages of entering data from a CRT is that the computer is able to check immediately the validity of the information. For instance, if the operator enters a letter for an AMOUNT, the computer will immediately reject the AMOUNT.

People who design computer systems have to be concerned about the human errors operators make. The computer experts have to program the machine to catch every error and force the operator to make an immediate correction. Let us consider an example.

Suppose the operator is to enter various changes for PATIENT 2222. The computer will display the following cue on the CRT Screen.

> **PATIENT NO.**

The operator should enter 2222. However, by mistake, the operator enters 1111.

Assume that the computer has been programmed to go to the patient's record and to display the patient's name. For example:

PATIENT NO.   1111   JOHN JONES   OK?

After displaying the patient's name, the computer waits for the operator to OK it.

Assume that the operator recognizes that there's been a mistake. The charge is really for FRED SMITH and not JOHN JONES. The operator enters "N" to indicate that JOHN JONES is not OK. The computer will then redisplay PATIENT NO., which gives the operator another chance to enter 2222 correctly.

Look at Figure 9-16.

The tall device contains the computer's memory, which is able to store numbers and letters. However, unlike a human brain, a computer's memory has limited capacity. For example, a large computer might be able to store 256,000 characters in memory. However, the patient's records for a 6,500-bed hospital will require millions of characters. Obviously, if a computer's memory can store a maximum of 256,000 characters,

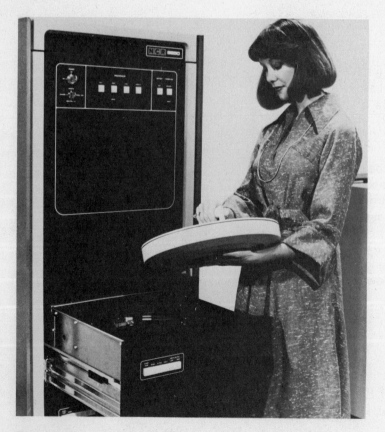

Figure 9-16. (*Courtesy of NCR Corporation, Dayton, Ohio.*)

it cannot keep all records in its memory at the same time. On the other hand, the computer needs to have access to all the information for every patient. In other words, the computer must have some way of storing the patient's records on file. Here is the solution.

Look again at Figure 9-16 and find the round case that the operator is holding in her hand.

This round case is known as a DISK PACK, and there is a disk inside the pack that looks like a long-playing record. However, instead of storing sounds, these disks store letters and numbers. Just as you might have a filing cabinet of patient's records on paper, the computer stores a file of patient's records on a disk pack. Disk packs come in various sizes. The pack in Figure 9-16 is able to store approximately 5 million characters. There are larger disk packs that can store 100 million characters.

Let us consider the kind of information that will be stored in the patient's record on the disk. Please scan Figure 9-17.

PATIENT'S ID NO.	NAME	SEX	DRUG ORDER					
			MON	DAY	YR	DOSAGE	TABLETS	DRUG
0000123	JOHN SMITH	M						

Figure 9-17. (Fictional—for training purposes only.)

Now let us find out what happens to the patient's record when a drug is ordered.

The form that the doctor fills out will be taken to the CRT, where the information will be entered on the keyboard. The computer will automatically write the drug order in the patient's record on the disk. It is important to note that whenever there is a new drug order, the computer will add the order to the patient's record on the disk.

One of the advantages of a computer is that it can print reports quickly. For example, some computers can print 3,000 lines per minute, which is like printing 60 pages in a minute.

REPORT FOR   WARD   003 –RUN ON 12–08–82   FOR DRUG ORDERS ACTIVE DURING THE PERIOD: NOV. 15.82 THROUGH DEC. 15.82

CLIENT'S NAME CONSEC. NO. PHYSICIAN'S NAME	DRUG CODE	NAME OF MEDICATION	DOSAGE PER ADMIN	FORM/ROUTE	FREQ.	DEC 01 08 15	PRESCRIPTION START DATE	STOP DATE	TOTAL CONSEC DAYS	7 DAY ADM	ORDER NUMBER
WASHINGTON, GEORGE, III											
3334445 35 YEAR OLD MALE											
DR. BROWN	50000	THORAZINE	50.00 MG	LIQ	QD	----------|------------|	DEC 06	DEC 15 82	408	8	12022
DR. BROWN	60000	MELLARIL	50.00 MG	TAB	BID	|------ |------*	DEC 06	DEC 11 82	7	8	34523
DR. RICHARDSON	50000	DILANTIN SOD	100.00 MG	CAP	PRN	------|---------*	DEC 04	DEC 10 82	30		12832
DR. BROWN	02000	VISTARIL	25.00 MG	LIQ	Q6H	----------------|	NOV 07	DEC 09 82	103	8	23822
DR. RICHARDSON	02000	NAVANE	1.00 MG	TAB	PRNHS	------------|	NOV 25	DEC 07 82	28		19814
DR. RICHARDSON	999991000	TEST DRUG X.X	500.00 MG	SUPP	BID	-------*	NOV 25	DEC 04 82	10		88881
DR. BROWN	999991020	TEST DRUG ZZ	500.00 MG	I.M.	TID		OCT 16	NOV 15 82	30		29433

Figure 9-18. (*Courtesy of Rockland Research Institute, Orangeburg, N.Y.*)

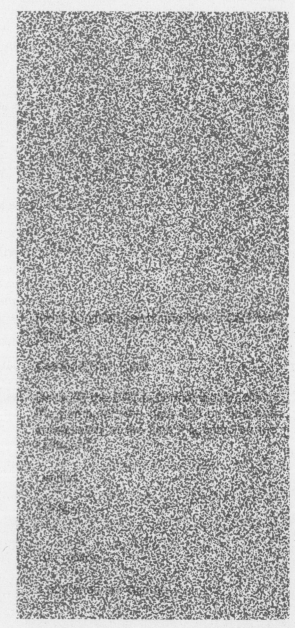

Scan the report on Figure 9-18.

Looking at this report you can see all the medication that has been ordered for WASHINGTON, GEORGE III.

Assume an average report of ten lines for each patient. Keep in mind that there are 6,500 beds at Rockland State Hospital. In that case, a total of 65,000 lines must be printed for this report. To give you an idea of the speed of a computer, assume that the computer prints 3,000 lines per minute. At that speed, the computer will print a 65,000-line report (for 6,500 patients) in less than one-half hour. Imagine trying to type the same report.

Review Questions

1. Name two methods of entering data into the computer.

2. What does CRT stand for?

3. With regard to the validity of the data being entered, what is the advantage of a CRT terminal over cards?

4. Does a computer have limited or unlimited memory?

5. How many characters can be stored on the disk pack shown in Figure 9-16?

6. How many characters can be stored on a large disk pack?

7. How many lines per minute can a fast computer print?

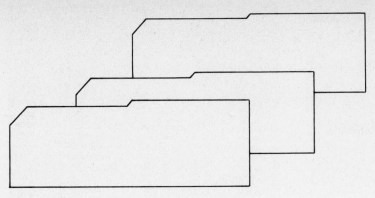

Figure 9-19.

What Is a Computer Program?

The computer's memory stores a series of instructions that tell the computer exactly what to do. You should remember that the series of instructions is called a program. Let us consider a simple example.

Notice the three cards in Figure 9-19.

Assume that you wish the computer to transfer the information in the cards to the patient's records on the disk. Let us consider what happens step by step.

The operator will place the cards in a special device known as a card reader (Figure 9-20).

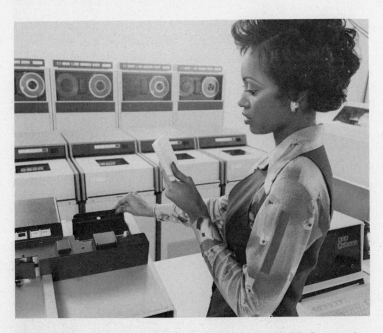

Figure 9-20. Use of a card reader. (*Courtesy of NCR Corporation, Dayton, Ohio.*)

Assume that the computer's memory is storing the following three instructions:

> **PROGRAM**
>
> **Step 1:   Read Card**
>
> **Step 2:   WRITE the information onto the Patient's Record on the disk**
>
> **Step 3:   Branch to Step 1**

Let's consider what the computer will do as it executes this program.

1. What does Step 1 instruct the computer to do?

As a result of executing Step 1, the computer will read the information from the first card into its memory.

2. What does Step 2 instruct the computer to do?

As a result of executing this step, the information about the patient that has been read in from the card will be transferred to the patient's record on the disk.

3. What does Step 3 instruct the computer to do?

As a result, the computer will go back to Step 1.

4. What does Step 1 instruct the computer to do?

As a result, the computer will read the information in the next card into its memory. This process will continue until the computer has transferred the information in all of the cards to the disk.

It should be noted that this program is an oversimplification. In actual fact, a computer program will be made up of hundreds and in some cases thousands of instructions. By the way, the people who write complex programs for computers are known as programmers.

Conclusion

As time goes on, computers are going to be installed in more and more hospitals and they are going to be used in innumerable ways.

Originally, computers were helpful for taking care of the business side of running a hospital. For instance, computers have been used to handle the patients' accounting records, for writ-

ing payroll checks, and for printing business reports. However, as you have seen in this chapter, computers can also be used to reduce the amount of time the doctor or nurse spends on the paperwork involved in ordering drugs.

Sometime soon, you may find computers being used at your hospital to read electrocardiograms. You may find that the devices that are used to analyze blood and urine samples are connected directly to the computer, which is able to type out a report immediately on the results of the tests.

No one really knows all the ways computers are going to be used in the future to help hospitals provide better service to their patients. However, as you can see, the possibilities are unlimited.

Unit One—Practice Tests

The following end-of-unit tests are designed to test your mastery of the subject matter in Chapters 1–9. There are four tests. Answers are provided for Tests 1 and 2, and the student should follow the usual Reinforced Learning procedures. Tests 3 and 4 are without answers and may be used in the classroom.

Unit One   Practice Test No. 1

1. If you gave $\frac{3}{5}$ of a 20-mg tablet, how many mg did you give?

2. If you used $2\frac{1}{2}$ tablets, 2 mg each, how much drug did you use?

3. To give 0.50 mg from 0.25-mg tablets, how many tablets should you use?

4. To give 7.5 mg from 15-mg tablets, how many tablets should you use?

5. If you need 2% of a 100-mg tablet, how much do you need?

6. What is $\frac{1}{3}$ % of 30?

7. 39.2°C equals how many degrees on the Fahrenheit scale?

8. 99.4°F equals how many degrees on the Celsius scale?

9. a) 5 g = _____ mg
   b) 2 kg = _____ g
   c) 500 ml = _____ liters

10. a) 10 pounds = _____ kg
    b) 140 cm = _____ in.
    c) 27 kg = _____ pounds

11. a) $\frac{1}{2}$ ml = _____ drops

    b) 2 teaspoonfuls = _____ ml
    c) 15 ml = _____ tablespoonfuls

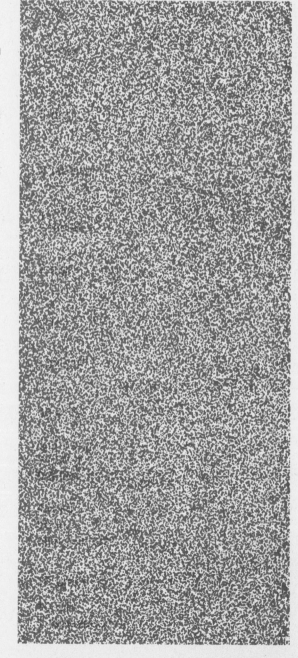

12. a) 200 mcg = _____ mg
    b) 0.075 mg = _____ mcg

13. $\dfrac{\frac{1}{500}}{\frac{1}{20}} = \dfrac{X}{1000}$. What does X equal?

14. $\dfrac{\frac{1}{10}}{1} = \dfrac{3}{X}$. What does X equal?

For each of the following orders, give the method and frequency of administration.

15. Give 250 mg tetracycline q.i.d.

16. Give 0.5 g Doriden h.s.

17. Give 10 mg Compazine IM, p.r.n.

18. Give 1 capsule Doxidan b.i.d.

19. Give 500 mg Diuril oral, q.d.

20. Give 25 mg Thorazine p.c.

Passing score is *0* errors.

Unit One   Practice Test No. 2

1. If you gave $\frac{3}{4}$ of a 250-mg tablet, how many mg did you give?

2. If you used 3 ampuls, 5-ml size, how many ml did you use?

3. To give codeine sulfate 15 mg from tablets 30 mg, use _____ tablets.

4. To give 15 ml from ampuls 5 ml, use _____ ampuls.

5. If you gave 1% of a 250-mg tablet, how many milligrams did you give?

6. What is $\frac{1}{4}$ % of 2 liters?

7. 38.2°C = _____ °F

8. 102.2°F = _____ °C

9. a) 146 pounds = _____ . kg
    b) 57 kg = _____ pounds

10. 138 cm = _____ in.

11. a) 4'11" = _____ cm
     b) 0.56 m = _____ cm

12. $\dfrac{\frac{1}{500}}{\frac{1}{100}} = \dfrac{X}{2,000}$ · Solve for X.

13. $\dfrac{\frac{2}{35}}{1} = \dfrac{2}{X}$ · Solve for X.

For each of the following orders, indicate the method and frequency of administration.

14. Give 1,000 mcg vitamin B_{12} IM, q.d.

15. Give 10 mg Librium p.r.n.

16. Give 100 mg Nembutal oral, h.s.

17. Give 15 mg Pro-Banthine a.c.

18. Give 15 cc Amphojel q.h.

19. a) 5 drops = _____ ml

     b) 30 ml = _____ tablespoonfuls
     c) 1 teaspoonful = _____ ml

20. 200 mg = _____ g

21. 1.3 kg = _____ g

22. 150 mcg = _____ mg

23. 3 kg = _____ lb

24. 0.05 mg = _____ mcg

25. 245 ml = _____ cc

Passing score is 0 errors.

Unit One   Practice Test No. 3

1. If you gave 20% of a 100-mg tablet, how many milligrams did you give? _____

2. If you gave $3\frac{1}{2}$ tablets, 3 mg each, how many milligrams did you give? _____

3. To give 0.3 mg of a drug from tablets 0.4 mg, how many tablets would you use? _____

4. To give aspirin 450 mg from tablets 300 mg, how many tablets would you use? _____

5. If you gave $\frac{1}{4}$ of a 10-ml ampul, how many ml did you give? _____

6. What is $\frac{1}{10}$ % of 5 g? _____ (answer in mg)

7. a) 200 pounds = _____ kg
   b) 86.4 kg = _____ pounds

8. 36.2°C = _____ °F

9. 96.8°F = _____ °C

10. a) 5'8" = _____ cm
    b) 140 cm = _____ in.

11. a) 2 g = _____ mg
    b) 37.5 cm = _____ m
    c) 381 ml = _____ liters

12. a) 5 drops = _____ ml
    b) 30 ml = _____ tablespoonfuls
    c) 2 teaspoonfuls = _____ ml

13. $\dfrac{\frac{1}{20}}{\frac{1}{2}} = \dfrac{X}{500}$ $X =$ _____

For each of the following orders, indicate the method and frequency of administration.

14. Give 100 mg Seconal h.s.

15. Give elixir of terpin hydrate 5 cc q.3h.

16. Give 0.5 g chlorothiazide q.a.m.

17. Give 35 U insulin subq, q.a.m.

18. Give 0.2 mg Ergotrate t.i.d.

19. 0.008 mg = _____ mcg

20. 350 mcg = _____ mg

Passing score is *0* errors.

Unit One   Practice Test No. 4

1. To give 125 mg of a drug from 250-mg tablets, how many tablets would you use? _____

2. To give $1\frac{1}{2}$ g from $\frac{3}{4}$-g tablets, how many tablets would you use? _____

3. If you gave $3\frac{1}{2}$ 15-mg tablets, how many milligrams did you give? _____

4. If you gave $\frac{1}{2}$ of a 7.5-mg tablet, how many milligrams did you give? _____

5. What is $\frac{1}{2}$ % of 100? _____

6. If you need 25% of a 150-mg tablet, how many milligrams do you need? _____

7. 41.8°C = _____ °F

8. 103.6°F = _____ °C

9. a) 275 mg = _____ g
   b) 185 cm = _____ m
   c) 185 km = _____ m

10. a) 250 pounds = _____ kg
    b) 100 kg = _____ pounds

11. a) 10 drops = _____ ml
    b) 45 ml = _____ tbsp
    c) 2 teaspoonfuls = _____ ml

12. 180 cm = _____ in.

13. 3'8" = _____ cm

14. $\dfrac{\frac{1}{50}}{X} = \dfrac{100}{5{,}000}$ $X =$ _____

15. a) 0.075 mg = _____ mcg
    b) 150 mcg = _____ mg

For each of the following orders, indicate the method and frequency of administration.

16. Give 10 mg morphine IM, p.r.n.

17. Give tetracycline 250 mg q.i.d.

18. Give 30 cc milk of magnesia h.s.

19. Give 15 cc aluminum hydroxide gel q.2h.

20. Give 500 mg aminophylline IV, stat.

Passing score is *0* errors.

Fractions of Tablets

Miscellaneous Medications and Procedures

Section 1

Read the following problem:

How many 20-mg tablets should be given to a patient who requires 40 mg?

Notice that the amount of the drug available in each tablet is 20 mg. The amount of the drug that is available in each tablet is called the available amount.

Notice that the amount of the drug we want to give the patient is 40 mg. The amount of the drug we want to give the patient is known as the desired amount.

Here is how to determine the number of tablets to give the patient.

$$\frac{\text{Desired amount}}{\text{Available amount}} = \text{Number of tablets}$$

Consider the following:

How many 75-mg tablets should be given for a total of 150 mg?

1. What is the desired amount?

2. What is the available amount?

3. Write the equation for determining the number of tablets to give to the patient.

4. Solve the equation.

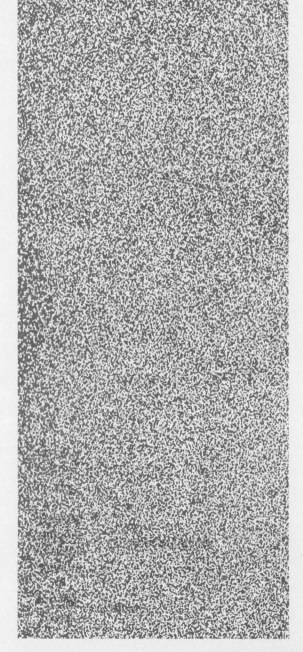

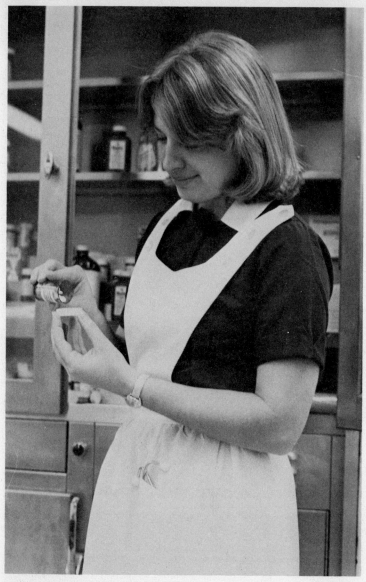

Figure 10-1. Student nurse pouring out a tablet. (*Courtesy of University of Illinois Hospitals, Chicago, Ill.*)

Note the following computer printout for a medication:

Name: ADAMS, HENRY	**RM–BD:** 227–A
Medication Order	**Available Medication**
SYNTHROID 0.3 MG	TABLETS 0.15 MG

5. What is the desired amount?

6. What is the available amount?

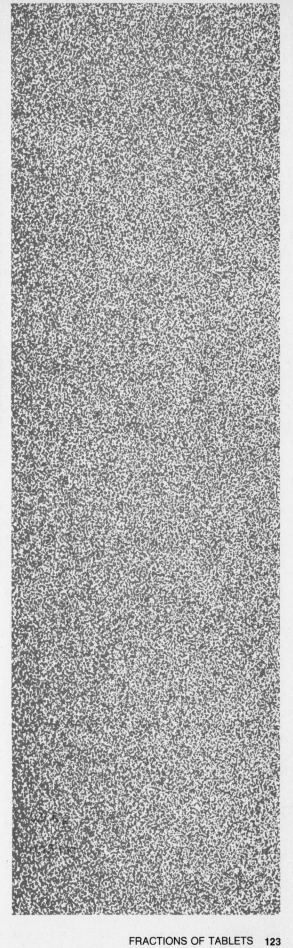

7. Write the equation for determining the number of tablets to give the patient.

8. Solve the equation.

Solve for the number of tablets in each of the following orders.

9. $\dfrac{.65}{.325} = 2$

Name: BLANC, ROSE	**RM–BD:** 118–2
Medication Order	**Available Medication**
ASPIRIN 0.65 G	TABLETS 0.325 G

10. $\dfrac{.4}{.4} = 1$

Name: KAUF, HELENE	**RM–BD:** 224–C
Medication Order	**Available Medication**
NITROGLYCERIN 0.4 MG	TABLETS 0.4 MG

11. $\dfrac{.5}{.25} = 2$

Name: COSTI, ARTURO	**RM–BD:** 349–1
Medication Order	**Available Medication**
DIGOXIN 0.5 MG	TABLETS 0.25 MG

12. $\dfrac{.5}{.25} = 2$

Name: ENGLISH, HENRY	**RM–BD:** 704–B
Medication Order	**Available Medication**
TERRAMYCIN 0.5 G	CAPSULES 0.25 G

13.

(handwritten: 500/250 = 2)

Name: KROLL, ANDREA	RM–BD: 915–3
Medication Order	**Available Medication**
TETRACYCLINE 500 MG	CAPSULES 250 MG

Passing score is no more than *1* error.

Section 2

Look at the following computer printout:

Name: KASSNER, GEORGE	RM–BD: 472–A
Medication Order	**Available Medication**
ASCORBIC ACID 0.5 G	TABLETS 500 MG

1. Write the equation to determine the number of tablets to give.

2. Substitute the known values.   *(handwritten: $\frac{.5\ g}{500\ mg}$)*

   Notice that the numerator is expressed in grams, and the denominator in milligrams. However, before we divide, both numerator and denominator must be expressed in the same units of measurement. Therefore, either convert grams to milligrams, or convert milligrams to grams.

3. How many milligrams equal 0.5 g?   *(handwritten: .5g × 1000 = 500 mg)*

4. Now solve for the number of tablets.   *(handwritten: $\frac{500\ mg}{500\ mg} = 1$)*

   That is one way to solve the problem. Let us consider another.

5. How many grams are in 500 mg?

   Therefore, in the above problem—

   $$\frac{0.5\ g}{500\ mg} = \frac{0.5\ g}{0.5\ g} = 1\ \text{tablet}$$

FRACTIONS OF TABLETS   125

Notice that the results are the same whether you change milligrams to grams, or grams to milligrams.

For very small amounts of medications, it is preferable to work in micrograms rather than milligrams.

Consider the following problem:

Name: ANDERSON, ARLENE	**RM–BD:** 302–1
Medication Order	**Available Medication**
DIGITOXIN 100 MCG	TABLETS 0.1 MG

6. Write the equation for determining the number of tablets to give the patient.

7. Substitute the known values. $\frac{100\,mcg}{.1\,mg}$

However, you cannot divide micrograms by milligrams. Therefore, you either have to change micrograms to milligrams or milligrams to micrograms.

For practice, let's try it both ways.

8. Change micrograms to milligrams and determine the number of tablets.

$$100\,mcg \times .001 = .1 \qquad \frac{.1}{.1} = 1$$
$$\frac{.001}{.100\,mg}$$

9. Let's solve the same equation using the second approach. Once again, write the equation with known values. $\frac{100\,mcg}{.1\,mg}$

10. Change milligrams to micrograms and determine the number of tablets.

$$.1\,mg \times 1000 = \frac{100\,mcg}{100\,mcg} = 1$$

As you can see, your answer should be the same whether you change milligrams to micrograms or vice versa. However, the preferred method is to change milligrams to micrograms.

Solve each of the following problems for the correct number of tablets.

11.

(handwritten: 30 mg = ½)
(handwritten: .06g × 1000 mg = 60 mg)

Name: KRAUS, ADOLF	RM–BD: 408–3
Medication Order	**Available Medication**
CODEINE 30 MG	TABLETS 0.06 G

12.

(handwritten: .3 × 1000 = 150/300 = ½)

Name: FLOWERS, LUCINDA	RM–BD: 873–A
Medication Order	**Available Medication**
SODIUM LEVOTHYROX- INE 150 MCG	TABLETS 0.3 MG

13.

(handwritten: .016g / .032g = ½)

Name: ODEN, CATHERINE	RM–BD: 370–2
Medication Order	**Available Medication**
CODEINE SULFATE 0.016 G	TABLETS 0.032 G

14.

(handwritten: 0.1 × 1000 = 100/50 = 2)

Name: AGREW, STAN	RM–BD: 338–A
Medication Order	**Available Medication**
ASCORBIC ACID 0.1 G	TABLETS 50 MG

15.

(handwritten: .15 × 1000 = 150/150 = 1)

Name: ANDREWS, JEANNE	RM–BD: 416–3
Medication Order	**Available Medication**
SYNTHROID 150 MCG	TABLETS 0.15 MG

16.

$.25 \times 1000 = \dfrac{250}{250} = 1$

Name: HYMAN, JEROME	RM–BD: 208–A
Medication Order	**Available Medication**
SERPASIL 0.25 MG	TABLETS 250 MCG

17.

$.25 \times 1000 = \dfrac{250}{500} = \dfrac{1}{2}$

Name: FRANK, MICHAEL	RM–BD: 1624–A
Medication Order	**Available Medication**
SULFISOXAZOLE 0.25 G	TABLETS 500 MG

Passing score is no more than *3* errors.

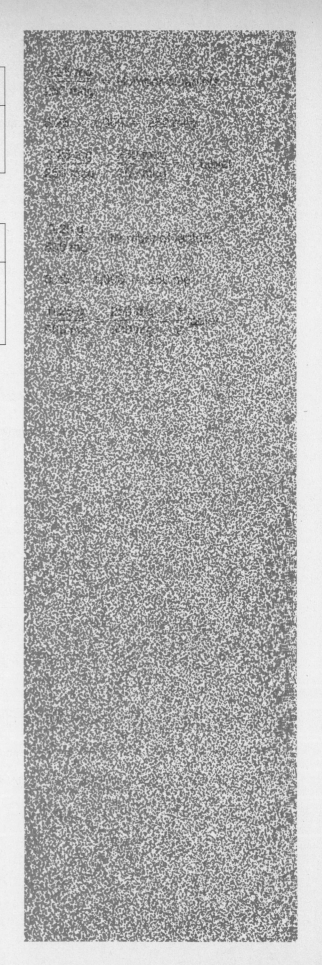

Chapter 11

Medications from Solutions

Section 1

Look at Figure 11-1 below:

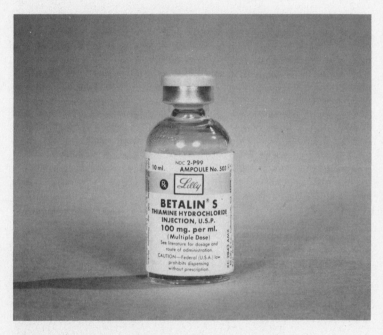

Figure 11-1. Vial of thiamine hydrochloride. (*Courtesy of Eli Lilly and Company, Indianapolis, Ind.*)

Notice that the label reads

100 mg per ml

This indicates that there are 100 mg of thiamine in 1 ml of the solution inside the ampul.

1. If you wanted to administer 200 mg, how many milliliters would you give the patient?

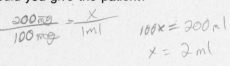

$$\frac{200\text{ mg}}{100\text{ mg}} = \frac{x}{1\text{ ml}} \qquad 100x = 200\text{ ml}$$
$$x = 2\text{ ml}$$

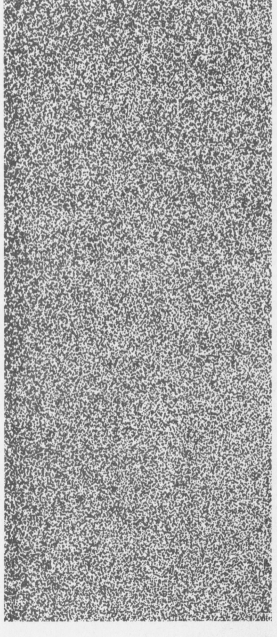

2. If you wanted to administer 25 mg, how many milliliters would you give the patient? $\frac{25\,mg}{100\,mg} = \frac{x}{1\,ml} = 100x = 25\,ml$

$x = .25\,ml$

$100\overline{)25.0}$

Frequently we have to administer a medication orally, intramuscularly (IM), or subcutaneously (subq) from a prepared solution. Therefore, we must know how to calculate the amount of solution to administer.

Here are a few points to know.

The amount of drug in a given volume of the medication is called the *available amount.* For instance, if the label reads 100 mg in 1 ml, the available amount is 100 mg.

Read the following label:

> sodium
> pentobarbital
>
> 100 mg/2 ml

3. What is the available amount? 100 mg

Select the available amount in each of the following:

4.

> vitamin B_{12}
>
> 1,000 mcg in 1 ml

5.

> 10% KCl
>
> 40 mEq in 30 ml

6.

> aminophylline
>
> 250 mg in 10 ml

7.

> heparin sodium
>
> 5,000 units/ml

In some hospitals, the order for a medication is written on a "medication card." The strength of the drug appears on the bottle. For example, consider the following medication card and vial:

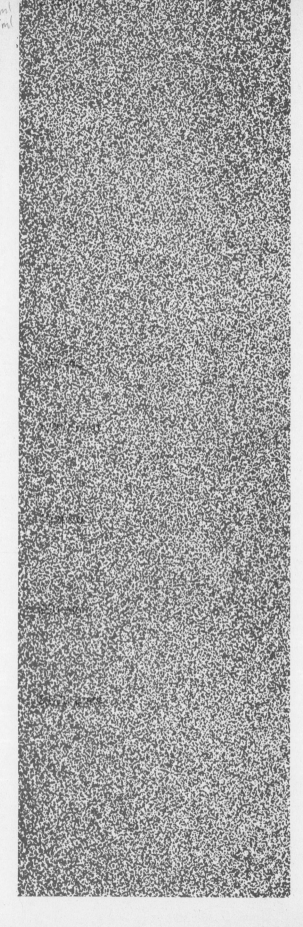

Name: Rosen, Henry   **Rm–Bd:** 409–1

codeine 30 mg subq stat

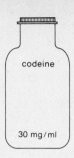

codeine

30 mg/ml

The medication card specifies an order for 30 milligrams of codeine to be given subcutaneously immediately. The bottle indicates that the strength of the drug is 30 milligrams per milliliter.

With the emphasis on computerization, more and more hospitals are using computer printouts to indicate the medication ordered, the frequency and method of administration, and the strength of the drug that is available. Consider the following printout:

Name: ROSEN, HENRY	**RM–BD:** 409–1
Medication Order	**Available Medication**
CODEINE 30 MG SUBQ STAT	30 MG/1 ML

Note that the computer printout provides the nurse with the same information as the card and vial.

We will use computer printouts for most of the medication orders in this book. However, the problems are solved exactly the same way when medication cards are used.

Reread the above printout.

The amount of drug ordered for the patient is called the *desired amount*.

For instance, if we are ordered to give the patient 30 mg codeine, the *desired amount* is 30 mg.

In each of the following problems, indicate the desired amount and the available amount.

8.

Name: BLACK, ARTHUR	**RM–BD:** 1817–A
Medication Order	**Available Medication**
CHLORAL HYDRATE 0.5 G WITH 1/2 GLASS WATER HS	500 MG/5 ML

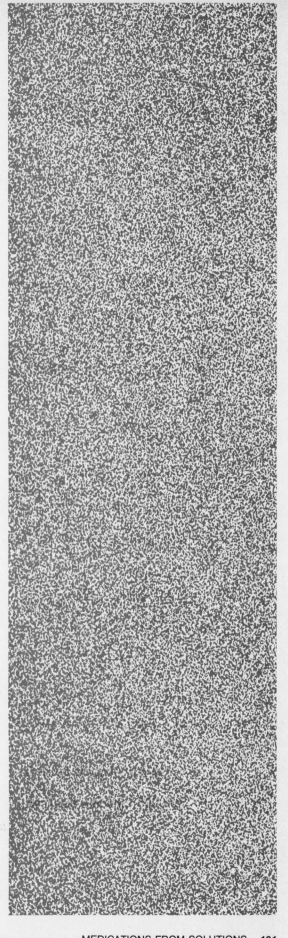

9.

Name: JOHNSON, PEARL	RM–BD: 325–B
Medication Order	**Available Medication**
MORPHINE SULFATE (A) 15 MG/1 ML (D) 7.5 MG IM PRN	

10.

Name: KARCH, MADELINE	RM–BD: 101–2
Medication Order	**Available Medication**
(D) 600,000 U PENICIL- LIN G PROCAINE IM STAT	(A) 300,000 U/1 ML

11.

Name: MCCLINTOCK, EVELYN	RM–BD: 558–B
Medication Order	**Available Medication**
DILAUDID (D) 2 MG IM Q4H	(A) 2 MG/1 ML

Passing score is no more than *1* error.

Section 2

Read the following computer printout:

Name: BURNS, RALPH	RM–BD: 967–2
Medication Order	**Available Medication**
VITAMIN K₁ 2.5 MG IM Q8H	1 MG/0.5 ML

1. What is the desired amount? 2.5 mg

2. What is the available amount? 1 mg

In this example, notice that 0.5 ml is on hand.

Assume that we must determine how much solution we are going to use.

Here is the equation for determining how much we are going to use.

$$\frac{\text{Desired amount}}{\text{Available amount}} = \frac{\text{How much we are going to use}}{\text{How much we have on hand}}$$

3. How much do we have on hand? .5ml

Note: *How much we have on hand is the amount of solution containing the available amount.* For example, in this case the printout indicates 1 mg/0.5 ml. Therefore, 0.5 ml is on hand.

4. Substitute the known values in the above equation.

$$\frac{2.5mg}{1mg} = \frac{x}{.5ml} \quad | \quad x = 1.25ml$$

There is one point that makes the setting up of this problem quite simple. That is, *the bottom half of the equation must repeat the strength indicated on the printout* (or on the label of the vial). In this example, the printout reads 1 mg/0.5 ml. The equation is:

$$\frac{\text{Desired amount}}{\text{Available amount}} = \frac{\text{How much we are going to use}}{\text{How much we have on hand}}$$

$$\frac{\text{Desired amount}}{1 \text{ mg}} = \frac{\text{How much we are going to use}}{0.5 \text{ ml}}$$

As you can see, the bottom half of the equation repeats the strength given on the printout.

5. Solve for how much we are going to use. x = 1.25ml

6. How is the medication to be administered? IM

7. How often is the medication to be administered? Q8H

Read the statement of the answer: To give Vitamin K_1 2.5 mg IM q.8h. from a vial labeled 1 mg/0.5 ml, withdraw 1.25 ml and administer intramuscularly every 8 hours.

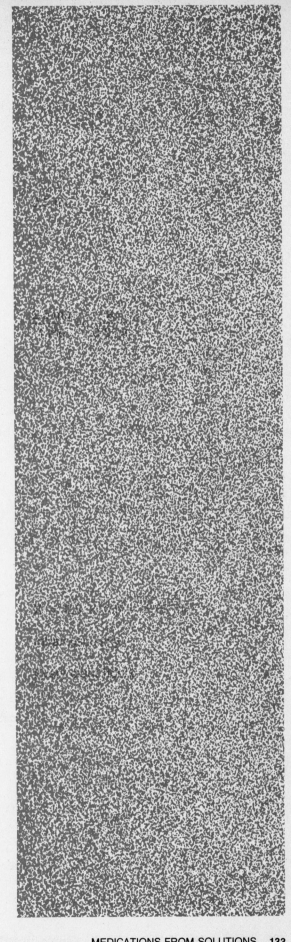

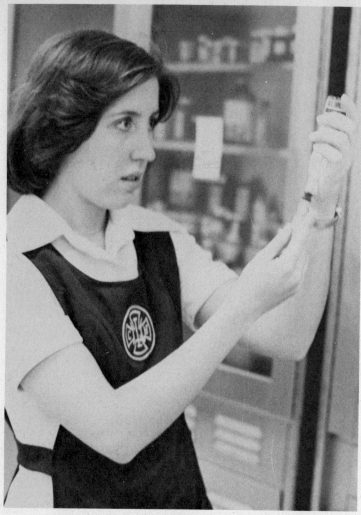

Figure 11-2. Student nurse withdrawing liquid medication from a vial. (*Courtesy of University of Illinois Hospitals, Chicago, Ill.*)

In each of the following problems, determine how much solution we are going to use, and write the statement of the answer.

8.

Name: BRENNAN, RUTH	RM–BD: 472–1
Medication Order	**Available Medication**
ASCORBIC ACID 100 MG IM BID	250 MG/1 ML

$$\frac{100 \text{ mg}}{250 \text{ mg}} = \frac{x}{1 \text{ ml}}$$

$$250x = 100 \text{ ml} \cdot 4$$

$$x = \frac{100 \cdot 8}{250}$$

$$x = .4 \text{ ml}$$

9.

Name: CALDER, SUSAN	RM–BD: 227–2
Medication Order	**Available Medication**
DEMEROL 80 MG IM Q3H	50 MG/1 ML

$$\frac{80mg}{50mg} = \frac{x}{1ml} \qquad 50x = 80ml$$

$$50\overline{)80} \qquad x = 1.6$$
$$\frac{30}{30}$$

10.

Name: ROGERS, JACQUELINE	RM–BD: 359–A
Medication Order	**Available Medication**
COMPAZINE 4MG IM Q4H	5 MG/1 ML

$$\frac{4mg}{5mg} = \frac{x}{1ml} \qquad 5x = 4ml$$
$$x = .8ml$$

11.

Name: WASSERMAN, MELVIN	RM–BD: 543–A
Medication Order	**Available Medication**
POTASSIUM CHLORIDE 20 MEQ BID	40 MEQ/30 ML

$$\frac{20\,mEq}{40\,mEq} = \frac{x}{30\,ml} \qquad 40x = 60ml$$

$$40\overline{)600} \qquad x = 1.5ml$$
$$\frac{4}{20}$$
$$\frac{}{20}$$

12.

Name: GOODMAN, ADELLE	RM–BD: 337–A
Medication Order	**Available Medication**
GANTRISIN 400 MG IM BID	2 G/5 ML

$$\frac{400mg}{2g} \times \frac{1g}{1000mg} \times \frac{5ml}{2} = 1.0$$

$$2g = 2 \times 1000 = 2000 \, mg$$

Bear in mind that before you can cross-multiply, you must either change 400 mg to grams or 2 g to milligrams. Since milligrams is the preferred unit for metric dosages, change grams to milligrams.

13.

Name: CANNEN, ESTHER	RM–BD: 427–2
Medication Order	**Available Medication**
TERRAMYCIN 75 MG IM Q8H	100 MG/2 ML

$$\frac{75mg}{100mg} \times 2ml = 1.50 \, ml$$

14.

Name: GORDON, BRUCE	RM–BD: 603–B
Medication Order	**Available Medication**
LANOXIN 250 MCG IM Q6H	0.5 MG/2 CC

$$\frac{250mcg}{.5mg} \times \frac{1mg}{1000mcg} \times 2cc = 1cc$$

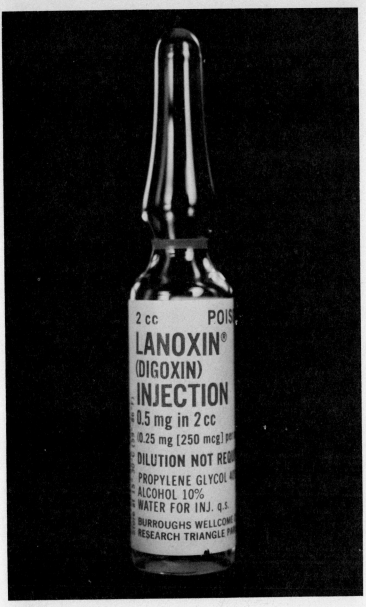

Figure 11-3. (*Photograph by Gail Shrader, Burroughs Wellcome Co., Research Triangle Park, North Carolina.*)

15.

Name: BILLINGS, GERTRUDE	RM–BD: 743–1
Medication Order	**Available Medication**
VASODILAN 7.5 MG IM BID	10 MG/2 ML

$$\frac{7.5\ mg}{10\ mg} \times 2\ ml = 1.5\ ml$$

Passing score is no more than *2* errors.

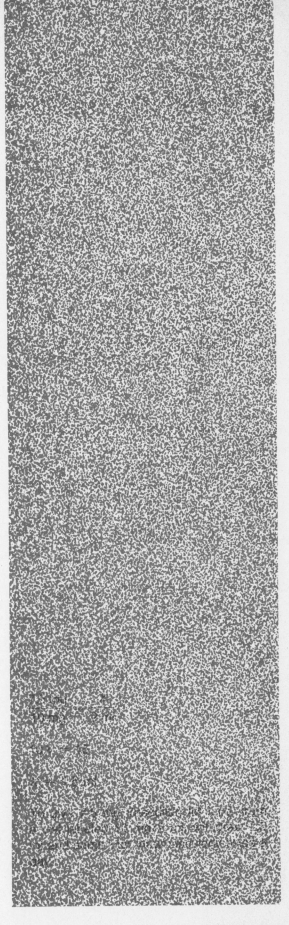

Section 3

Read the following printout:

Name: BLACK, ERMALINE	**RM–BD:** 600–A
Medication Order	**Available Medication**
MAGNESIUM SULFATE, 20 G PO	50%

Here again, to solve the problem, we want to use the same formula, where the lower half repeats the strength of the available medication. However, notice that the printout reads:

50%

50% means . . . . 50 g in 100 ml.

Consider the following printout:

Name: CUTTER, HEATHER	**RM–BD:** 103–B
Medication Order	**Available Medication**
DEXTROSE 25 G PO	1:4

Please note that 1:4 is understood to mean 1 g in 4 ml.

In each of the following problems, determine how much of the drug we are going to use and write the statement of the answer.

1.

Name: ALBION, REGIS	**RM–BD:** 228–1
Medication Order	**Available Medication**
EPINEPHRINE 0.5 MG SUBQ STAT	1:1,000

$$\frac{.5 \, mg}{1 \, g} = \frac{x}{1,000 \, ml}$$

$$1 \, g = 1000 \, mg$$

$$\frac{0.5 \, mg}{1000 \, mg} = \frac{x}{1000 \, ml} \qquad 1000x = 500 \, ml$$

$$x = 0.5 \, ml$$

2.

Name: VITALI, TERESA	**RM–BD:** 339–B
Medication Order	**Available Medication**
MAGNESIUM SULFATE 500 MG IM QD	50%

$$\frac{500\,mg}{50\,g} = \frac{x}{100\,ml}$$

$$\frac{500\,mg}{50,000\,mg} = \frac{x}{100\,ml}$$

$$50,000\,x = 50,000\,ml \qquad x = 1\,ml$$

3.

Name: GRANT, JEAN	**RM–BD:** 404–1
Medication Order	**Available Medication**
GARAMYCIN 80 MG IM Q8H	40 MG/1 ML

$$\frac{80\,mg}{40\,mg} = \frac{x}{1\,ml}$$

$$40\,x = 80\,ml \qquad x = 2\,ml$$

4.

Name: KRAFT, ANDREA	**RM–BD:** 573
Medication Order	**Available Medication**
ISUPREL 0.2 MG SUBQ BID	1:5,000

$$\frac{.2\,mg}{1\,g} = \frac{x}{5,000\,ml}$$

$$\frac{.2\,mg}{1000\,mg} = \frac{x}{\frac{5000\,ml}{\frac{.2}{1000}}}$$

$$1000\,x = 1000\,ml$$

$$x = 1\,ml$$

5.

Name: PRICE, HENRY	RM–BD: 328–A
Medication Order	**Available Medication**
POTASSIUM CHLORIDE 3 G BID	10%

$$\frac{3g}{10g} = \frac{x}{100\,ml}$$

$$10x = 300\,ml \qquad x = 30\,ml$$

6.

Name: DOUGLAS, JACK	RM–BD: 482–2
Medication Order	**Available Medication**
THIAMINE HYDROCHLORIDE 50 MG IM BID	100 MG/1 ML

$100\overline{)50.0}$ .50

$$\frac{50\,mg}{100\,mg} = \frac{x}{1\,ml}$$

$$100x = 50\,ml \qquad x = .5\,ml$$

7.

Name: PRENTICE, SYLVIA	RM–BD: 600
Medication Order	**Available Medication**
VITAMIN B$_{12}$ 250 MCG IM QD	1,000 MCG/1 ML

$$\frac{250\,mcg}{1,000\,mcg} = \frac{x}{1\,ml}$$

$$1000x = 250\,ml \qquad x = .25\,ml$$

8.

Name: O'NEAL, MARY	RM–BD: 330–B
Medication Order	**Available Medication**
DILAUDID 1.5 MG IM Q4H	2 MG/1 ML

$2\overline{)1.50}$ .75
14
10

$$\frac{1.5\,mg}{2\,mg} = \frac{x}{1\,ml}$$

$$2x = 1.5\,ml$$

$$x = .75\,ml$$

9.

Name: BLACKWOOD, JEANNE	RM–BD: 109–1
Medication Order	**Available Medication**
DEMEROL 100 MG IM Q4H	50 MG/1 ML

$$\frac{100\ mg}{50\ mg} = \frac{x}{1\ ml}$$

$$50x = 100\ ml \qquad x = 2\ ml$$

10.

Name: LITTLE, LEWIS	RM–BD: 449–A
Medication Order	**Available Medication**
EPINEPHRINE 0.5 MG SUBQ STAT	1:1,000

$$\frac{.5\ mg}{1\ g} = \frac{x}{1000\ ml}$$

$$\frac{.5\ mg}{1000\ mg} = \frac{x}{1000\ ml}$$

$$1000x = 500\ ml \qquad x = .5\ ml$$

11.

Name: MCDONOUGH, PAT	RM–BD: 204–2
Medication Order	**Available Medication**
PANHEPRIN 8,000 U SUBQ Q8H	5,000 U/1 ML

$$\frac{8000\ U}{5000\ U} = \frac{x}{1\ ml}$$

$$5000x = 8000\ ml$$

$$x = 1.6\ ml$$

$$5\overline{)8.0} \quad 1.6$$

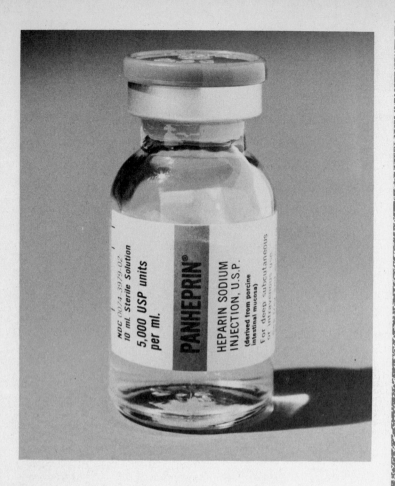

12.

Name: HALPRIN, KATHY	**RM–BD:** 112–3
Medication Order	**Available Medication**
TETRACYCLINE 500 MG BID	125 MG/5 CC

$$\frac{500\,mg}{125\,mg} = \frac{x}{5cc}$$

$$125x = 2500cc \qquad x = 20cc$$

13.

Name: STAFFORD, ERIC	**RM–BD:** 230–4
Medication Order	**Available Medication**
MORPHINE SULFATE 10 MG SUBQ STAT	15 MG/1 ML

$$\frac{10\,mg}{15\,mg} = \frac{x}{1ml}$$

$$15x = 10ml \qquad x = .67ml$$

Passing score is no more than *3* errors.

12

Infants' and Children's Dosages

Because infants and children require smaller dosages than adults, it is important for us to know how to determine pediatric dosages. The most accurate method specifies the dosage in terms of the amount of drug that should be administered in 24 hours per kilogram of a child's weight. For example, the label on a vial reads—

> cephradine
>
> for injection
>
> pediatric dosage for children: 50 mg/kg/day in equally divided doses

This *means* that 50 milligrams of cephradine should be given by injection for each kilogram of a child's weight. The medication is to be administered in equally divided doses over a period of 24 hours.

Another vial might read:

> erythromycin
>
> for oral use
>
> pediatric dosage for infants under 4.5 kg: 40 mg/kg/day in divided doses

This means that infants weighing less than 4.5 kilograms should be given 40 milligrams of erythromycin daily for each kilogram of the baby's weight. The medication is to be administered orally in divided doses.

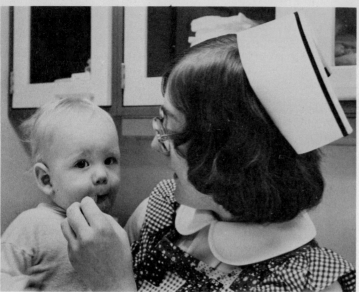

Figure 12-1. Infant receiving medication. (*Courtesy of School of Nursing, St. Francis Hospital, Evanston, Ill.*)

Section 1 Pediatric Dosages

Assume that you must determine the dosage for an infant weighing 10 kg. The following label appears on the vial—

> pediatric dosage
>
> 75 mg/kg/day

To determine the pediatric dosage that should be administered in 24 hours, multiply the dosage on the label by the weight of the child.

For example,

$$75 \text{ mg/kg} \times 10 \text{ kg} = 750 \text{ mg}$$

This means that the child should receive 750 mg in 24 hours.

1. The pediatric dosage of a drug is 50 mg/kg/day. How much medication should be given to an infant weighing 10 kg in 24 hours?

2. The pediatric dosage of a drug is 100 mg/kg/day. How much should be administered to a 20-kg child during a 24-hour period?

Consider the following—

Give disodium carbenicillin q.6h. IM to a child weighing 15 kg. The label on the vial reads: pediatric dosage 100 mg/kg/day. Determine the appropriate dosage that should be given to a child each time the drug is administered.

Step 1

Multiply the pediatric dosage on the label by the weight of the child to determine the dosage to be administered in 24 hours.

$$100 \text{ mg/kg} \times 15 \text{ kg} = 1{,}500 \text{ kg}$$

Step 2

Determine the number of time periods per day.

Since q.6h. means every 6 hours, the drug will be administered 4 times in 24 hours.

Step 3

Divide the dosage you found in Step 1 by the number of time periods in Step 2. The result is the amount to be given per dose.

$$1{,}500 \div 4 = 375 \text{ mg}$$

For each of the following problems, calculate—

The total amount of the drug that should be administered in 24 hours.

The number of doses in 24 hours.

The amount of each dose.

3. Give disodium carbenicillin q.4h. IM to a child weighing 15 kg.

> disodium carbenicillin
>
> pediatric dosage
>
> 100 mg/kg/day

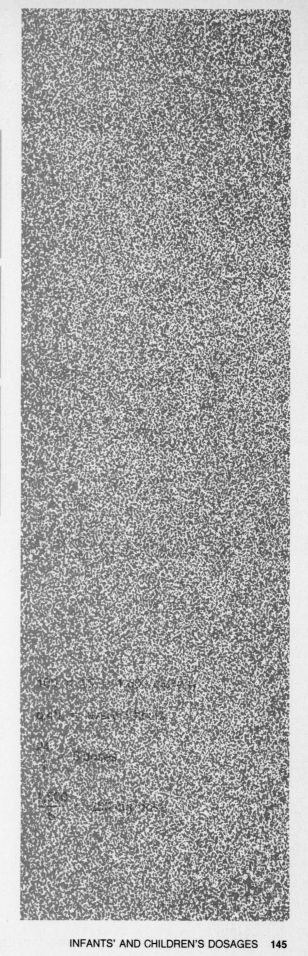

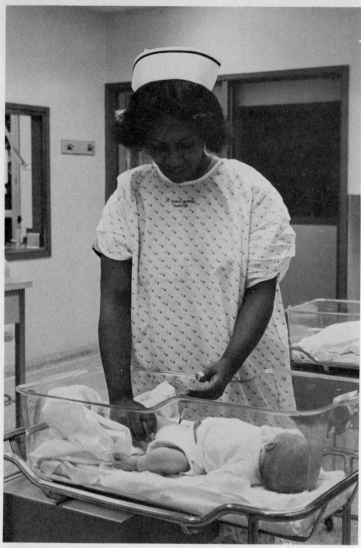

Figure 12-2. Administering an injection to an infant. (*Courtesy of School of Nursing, St. Francis Hospital, Evanston, Ill.*)

4. Give ticarcillin q.4h. IM to an infant weighing 6 kg.

> ticarcillin
>
> pediatric dosage
>
> 600 mg/kg/day

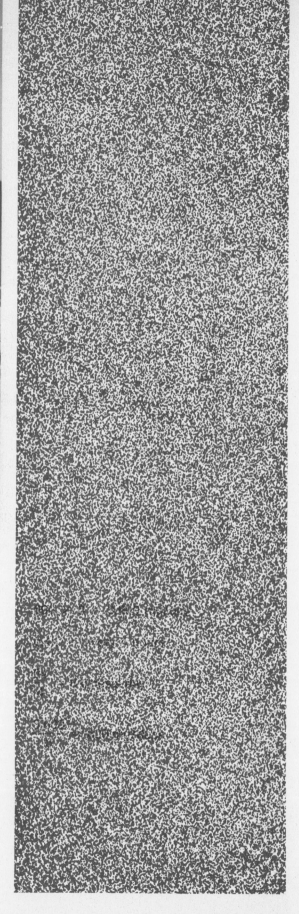

5. Give cephradine q.i.d. IM to a child weighing 12 kg.

```
┌─────────────────────────┐
│                         │
│       cephradine        │
│                         │
│     pediatric dosage    │
│                         │
│      50 mg/kg/day       │
│                         │
└─────────────────────────┘
```

6. Give sodium ampicillin t.i.d. IM to a child weighing 30 kg.

```
┌─────────────────────────┐
│                         │
│     sodium ampicillin   │
│                         │
│     pediatric dosage    │
│                         │
│      30 mg/kg/day       │
│                         │
└─────────────────────────┘
```

7. Give tetracycline hydrochloride b.i.d. IV to a child weighing 25 kg.

```
┌───────────────────────────────┐
│                               │
│   tetracycline hydrochloride  │
│                               │
│       pediatric dosage        │
│                               │
│        12 mg/kg/day           │
│                               │
└───────────────────────────────┘
```

8. Give sodium methicillin q.i.d. IM to an infant weighing 8 kg.

```
┌─────────────────────────┐
│                         │
│    sodium methicillin   │
│                         │
│     pediatric dosage    │
│                         │
│      100 mg/kg/day      │
│                         │
└─────────────────────────┘
```

Passing score is no more than *2* errors.

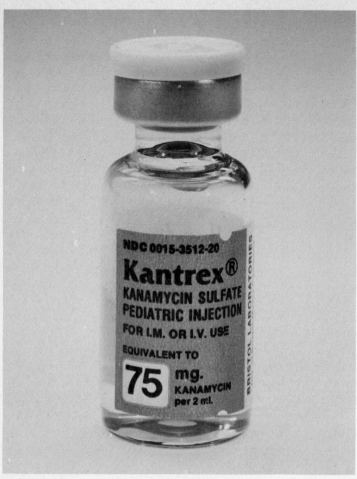

Consider the following:

Name: CORTEZ, JUANITA	RM–BD: 100–4
Wt. in kg. 5.0	

Medication Order	Available Medication
KANTREX IM Q6H	75 MG/2 ML

Pediatric Dosage
15 MG/KG/DAY

9. How much Kantrex should be given to the patient in one day?

10. How much Kantrex should be administered every 6 hours?

11. How is the medication to be administered?

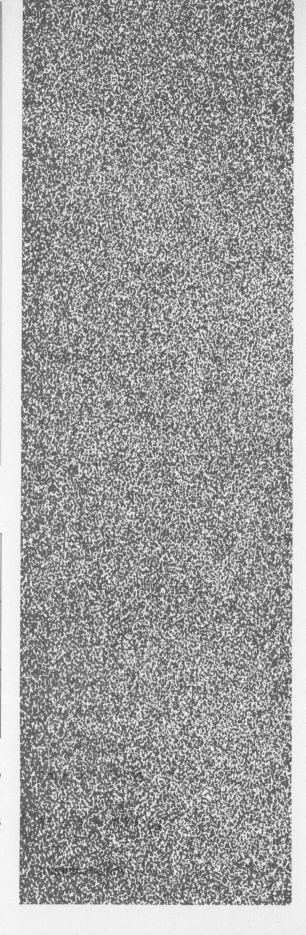

12. Assume that you want to determine the number of milliliters to administer per individual dose. What equation would you use?

13. Substitute the known values and calculate the amount of Kantrex to use per individual dose.

14. Try to write the appropriate statement.

Look at the following order.

Name: RODREQUEZ, TONY	**RM–BD:** 239–3
Wt. in kg. 8.0	

Medication Order	Available Medication
GARAMYCIN IM Q8H	10 MG/1.0 ML

Pediatric Dosage
7.5 MG/KG/DAY

15. Assume that you wish to determine the number of ml per dose. What is the first thing you need to calculate?

16. How should you determine the mg to administer per day?

17. Determine the mg to administer per day.

18. What is the next thing you must determine?

19. How many times is the dose to be administered?

20. What is the next thing to determine?

21. Calculate the mg per dose.

22. What equation should you use to determine the number of ml to use?

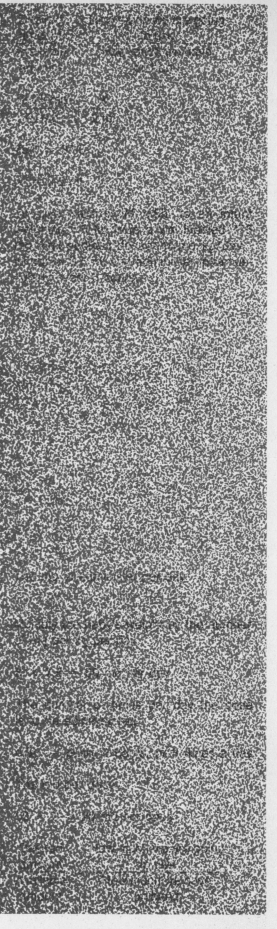

23. Substitute and solve the equation.

24. Write the appropriate statement.

For each of the following problems, calculate the amount of medication per dose and write a statement of your answer.

25.

Name: KANTCHELL, LOUIS	**RM–BD:** 123–D
Wt. in kg. 20.0	

Medication Order	Available Medication
VELOSEF Q12H	250 MG/5 ML

Pediatric Dosage
25/MG/KG/DAY

26. If this medication is to be taken at home, how much medication should be administered to the child every 12 hours?

27.

Name: EVANS, CAROLYN	**RM–BD:** 220–1
Wt. in kg. 15.0	
Medication Order	**Available Medication**
OMNIPEN Q8H	125 MG/5 ML
Pediatric Dosage	
100 MG/KG/DAY	

15 × 100 = 1,500 mg/day

q8h = every 8 hours, or 3 times a day

1,500 ÷ 3 = 500 mg per dose

$$\frac{500 \text{ mg}}{125 \text{ mg}} = \frac{X}{5 \text{ ml}}$$

125X = 2,500

X = 20 ml

To give Omnipen q8h to a child weighing 15.0 kg from a vial labeled "125 mg/5 ml, pediatric dosage 100 mg/kg/day," pour out 20 ml and administer orally every 8 hours.

28.

Name: ANDERSON, ALVIN	**RM–BD:** 303–2
Wt. in kg. 40.0	
Medication Order	**Available Medication**
TETRACYCLINE Q6H	125 MG/5 ML
Pediatric Dosage	
25 MG/KG/DAY	

40 × 25 = 1,000 mg per day

q6h = every 6 hours, or 4 times a day

1,000 ÷ 4 = 250 mg per dose

$$\frac{250 \text{ mg}}{125 \text{ mg}} = \frac{X}{5 \text{ ml}}$$

125X = 1,250

X = 10 ml

To give tetracycline q6h to a child weighing 40.0 kg from a vial labeled "125 mg/5 ml, pediatric dosage 25 mg/kg/day," pour out 10 ml and administer orally every 6 hours.

29.

Name: O'BRIEN, CHARLES	**RM–BD:** 111–A
Wt. in kg. 10.0	

Medication Order	**Available Medication**
KANAMYCIN SULFATE IM BID	75 MG/2 ML

Pediatric Dosage
15 MG/KG/DAY

Passing score is no more than *1* error.

Chapter 13

Insulin Dosage

Section 1

Look at the following illustration.

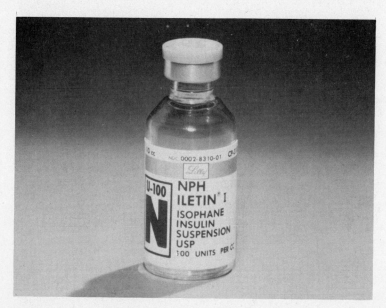

Figure 13-1. Bottle of U-100 insulin. (*Courtesy of Eli Lilly and Company, Indianapolis, Ind.*)

Notice the label "U-100."

U-100 (U100) indicates that there are 100 units of insulin per 1 ml (or 1 cc) of solution.

An increasing number of medications (e.g., insulin, penicillin, etc.) are given in units rather than in other terms of measurement. One of the most common of these is insulin, which comes in bottles labeled U-100. The designation U-100 tells us there are 100 units of insulin present in 1 ml (or 1 cc) of solution.

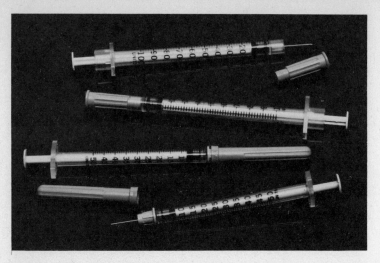

Figure 13-2. Disposable insulin syringes. (*Courtesy of Becton-Dickinson, Rutherford, N.J.*)

Insulin is generally given by means of an insulin syringe, which is graduated directly in units.

Name: HENRY, MAURICE	**RM–BD:** 338-2
Medication Order	**Available Medication**
INSULIN 30 UNITS SUBQ QAM	100 U/1 ML

If you want to give an injection of 30 units of U-100 insulin, withdraw the insulin in the U-100 syringe until the level of the liquid reaches the 30 mark on the scale.

Notice the following illustration.

Sometimes, an insulin syringe is not available, and we must use a tuberculin syringe to administer the insulin.

Let us now find out how to administer insulin using the tuberculin syringe.

Look at the above order for 30 units of insulin. How may this be administered using a tuberculin syringe?

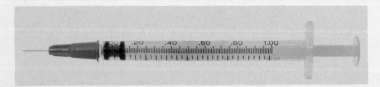

Figure 13-3. Tuberculin syringe with needle. (*Courtesy of Becton-Dickinson, Rutherford, N.J.*)

Here is the formula to use.

$$\frac{\text{Desired amount}}{\text{Available amount}} = \frac{\text{How much we are going to use}}{\text{How much we have on hand}}$$

Again, in using this formula, the bottom half should agree with the label on the bottle.

1. In the above instruction, what is the desired amount?

Bear in mind that the bottle of insulin contains 100 units in 1 ml of solution.

2. What is the available amount?

3. Substitute the value you know, and solve for how much of the solution we are going to use.

Therefore, we are going to use 0.30 ml of U-100 insulin.

Read the statement of the answer:

To give 30 units of insulin withdraw 0.30 ml of U-100 insulin and administer subcutaneously every morning.

In each of the following problems, solve for the amount of U-100 insulin to give the patient and write a statement of your answer.

4. How many milliliters of insulin are needed to give 45 units?

5. How many milliliters of insulin are needed to give 60 units?

6. How many milliliters of insulin are needed to give 36 units?

Passing score is *0* errors.

Chapter 14

Medications from Powders

Many medications are unstable when stored in solution and so are packed in powder (or granular) form in a vial. If the medication is stored as a powder (or as granules), it must be dissolved before use.

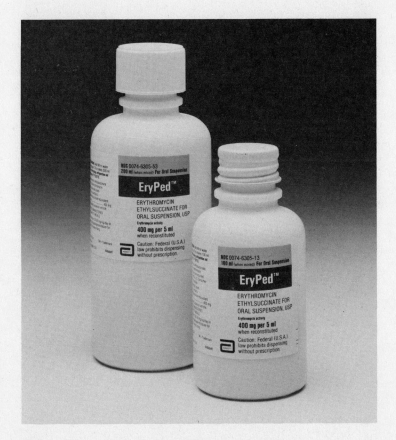

Figure 14-1. Granular medication—to be dissolved before use. (*Courtesy of Abbott Laboratories, North Chicago, Ill.*)

When a medication is stored as a powder in a vial, the powder usually takes up appreciable volume. In these cases, the bottles or package inserts are clearly labeled to show the amount of sterile diluent to add to or inject into the vial.

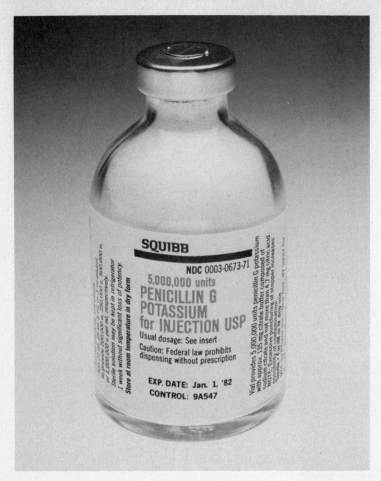

Figure 14-2. (*Courtesy of E. R. Squibb & Sons, Princeton, New Jersey.*)

For example, the label shows the amount of medication in the powder:

The package insert usually provides the nurse with directions for diluting the powder with a sterile diluent.

> Directions for reconstitution:
>
> 5,000,000 units—add 23 ml sterile water
> to provide 200,000 units/1.0 ml

Notice that the directions instruct the nurse to add 23 ml sterile water to the vial containing 5,000,000 U penicillin in order to yield a reconstituted solution that contains 200,000 units of penicillin per milliliter. Assume the following printout:

Name: MARTINEZ, CARLOS	RM–BD: 116–2

Medication Order	Available Medication
PENICILLIN 400,000 U IM Q4H	5,000,000 U

Directions for reconstitution

ADD 23 ML STERILE WATER TO PROVIDE 200,000 U/1.0 ML.

You have already learned the formula for determining how much of the solution to use.

$$\frac{\text{Desired amount}}{\text{Available amount}} = \frac{\text{How much we are going to use}}{\text{How much we have on hand}}$$

According to the directions on the insert, after 23 ml of sterile water have been added, the vial will contain 200,000 units/1.0 ml. The printout specifies that 400,000 U are to be administered. The nurse's task is to determine the number of ml of the diluted solution to use.

In this problem, the desired amount is 400,000 U, the available amount is 200,000 U, the amount we are going to use is X, and the amount we have on hand is 1 ml.

Then, inserting these figures in the formula:

$$\frac{400,000 \text{ U}}{200,000 \text{ U}} = \frac{X}{1 \text{ ml}}$$

$$200,000X = 400,000$$

$$X = 2 \text{ ml}$$

Here's an important concept to bear in mind. The insert specifies the reconstituted strength as 200,000 U/1.0 ml. In the formula that you have learned, *the values below the line should always agree with the reconstituted strength on the insert.* In the above equation, notice that the values below the line are the same as the reconstituted strength on the insert (200,000 U/1.0 ml).

Where sterile water is added to the powder in a vial, many solutions are stable for only short periods of time. Therefore, the nurse should not prepare them until they are needed. After they are prepared, the nurse must relabel, indicating the time and date of preparation as well as the amount of medication per milliliter. In the above problem the vial must be relabeled. The statement is:

To give 400,000 U penicillin IM q.4h. from a vial labeled "5,000,000 units—Directions for reconstitution: add 23 ml sterile water to yield a solution that contains 200,000 units/1.0 ml," inject 23 ml sterile water into the vial, shake until dissolved, withdraw 2 ml, and administer IM every 4 hours. Relabel the vial with the date and time of preparation. Also write "200,000 U/1.0 ml" on the label.

Note: After preparing the solution, the nurse must always write the number of units of medication per milliliter on the label. For example, in the previous problem, the new label must show 200,000 U/1.0 ml. The number of units per milliliter you write on the label should be the same as the concentration given in the directions for reconstitution.

Let's consider several problems.

Look at the following printout:

Name: METROPOLIS, GEORGE	**RM–BD:** 209–1

Medication Order	**Available Medication**
STAPHCILLIN 750 MG IM QD 10 A.M.	1.0 G

Directions for reconstitution

ADD 1.5 ML STERILE WATER. EACH 1.0 ML WILL CONTAIN APPROXIMATELY 500 MG STAPHCILLIN. SOLUTION IS STABLE AT ROOM TEMPERATURE FOR 24 HOURS.

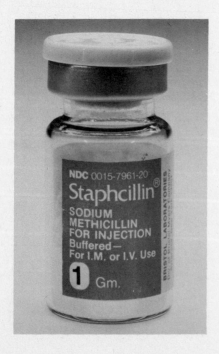

1. What is the desired amount? 750mg

2. What is the available amount? 500mg

3. What is the amount we are going to use? x

4. What is the amount we have on hand? 1ml

5. Use the following formula to determine how much we are going to use.

$$\frac{\text{Desired amount}}{\text{Available amount}} = \frac{\text{How much we are going to use}}{\text{How much we have on hand}}$$

$$\frac{750mg}{500mg} = \frac{x}{1ml} \quad 500x = 750ml \quad x = 1.5ml$$

The directions on the insert indicate that the reconstituted solution is to contain 500 mg/1.0 ml. Note that the values in the bottom half of the equation repeat the concentration of the reconstituted solution.

The statement is:

To give Staphcillin 750 mg IM q.d. 10 A.M. from a vial labeled "1.0 g: Directions for reconstitution—add 1.5 ml sterile water. Each 1.0 ml will contain approximately 500 mg Staphcillin," inject 1.5 ml sterile water, shake until dissolved, withdraw 1.5 ml, and administer intramuscularly at 10 A.M. every morning.

Note that since such a small volume is left, the remainder is discarded and does not have to be relabeled.

Let us consider another example.

Name: SAUNDERS, BARBARA	**RM–BD:** 225–A

Medication Order	**Available Medication**
GEOPEN 1 G IM Q6H	5 G

Directions for reconstitution

ADD 7.0 ML STERILE WATER TO YIELD A SOLUTION THAT CONTAINS 1 G/2 ML. RECONSTITUTED SOLUTION IS STABLE FOR 24 HOURS AT ROOM TEMPERATURE.

6. What is the desired amount? 1G

7. What is the available amount? 1G

8. What is the amount we are going to use? x

9. What is the amount we have on hand? 2ml

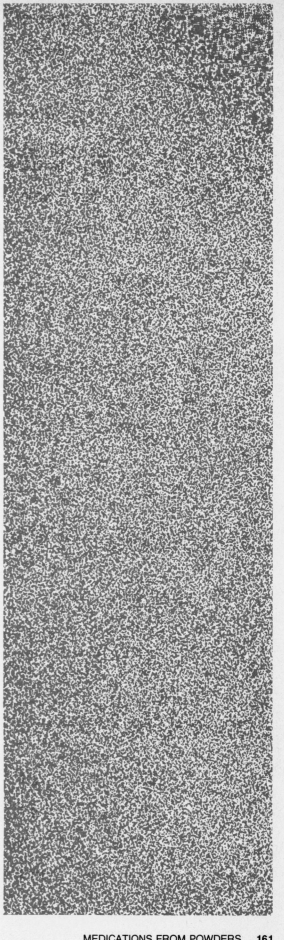

10. Using the formula, determine how much we are going to use.

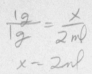

$$\frac{1g}{1g} = \frac{x}{2ml}$$

$$x = 2ml$$

The statement is:

To give Geopen 1 g IM q.6h. from a vial labeled "5 g— Directions for reconstitution: add 7.0 ml of sterile water to yield a solution that contains 1 g/2 ml. Reconstituted solution is stable for 24 hours at room temperature," add 7.0 ml of sterile water to the vial, shake until dissolved, withdraw 2 ml, and administer intramuscularly every 6 hours. Relabel the vial "1 g/2 ml" and also label date and time of preparation.

In each of the following problems, calculate the amount of medication to be given and write the proper statement.

1.

Name: MCCANN, JULIET	RM–BD: 904–2

Medication Order	Available Medication
AMPICILLIN 500 MG QID	100 ML VIAL

Directions for reconstitution

ADD 66 ML WATER. RECONSTITUTED SOLUTION WILL CONTAIN 125 MG/5 ML. SHAKE WELL BEFORE USING. SOLUTION IS STABLE FOR 7 DAYS AT ROOM TEMPERATURE AND FOR 14 DAYS UNDER REFRIGERATION.

$$\frac{500\,mg}{125\,mg} = \frac{x}{5ml}$$

$$125x = 2500ml$$

$$x = 20ml$$

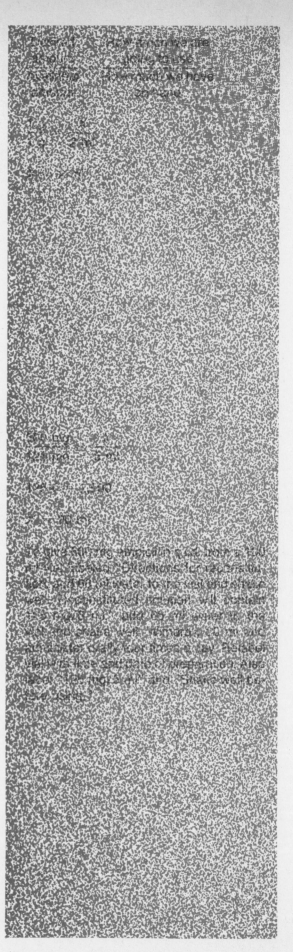

2.

Name: HOOVER, DAVID	**RM–BD:** 314–B

Medication Order	**Available Medication**
PENICILLIN G 250,000 U IM Q4H	5,000,000 U

Directions for reconstitution

ADD 18 ML STERILE WATER TO PROVIDE A CONCENTRATION OF 250,000 U/1.0 ML. RECONSTITUTED SOLUTION IS STABLE FOR 1 WEEK UNDER REFRIGERATION.

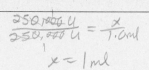

$$\frac{250,000\ U}{250,000\ U} = \frac{x}{1.0\ ml}$$

$$x = 1\ ml$$

3.

Name: OLSEN, RALPH	**RM–BD:** 1215–1

Medication Order	**Available Medication**
GEOPEN 0.5 G IM Q6H	2 G

Directions for reconstitution

ADD 4 ML STERILE WATER TO YIELD A CONCENTRATION OF 1 G/2.5 ML. SOLUTION IS STABLE AT ROOM TEMPERATURE FOR 24 HOURS.

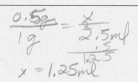

$$\frac{0.5g}{1g} = \frac{x}{\frac{2.5ml}{1.25}}$$

$$x = 1.25\ ml$$

4.

Name: MALONE, LAVINIA	**RM–BD:** 107–C

Medication Order	**Available Medication**
STREPTOMYCIN IM: 1 G BID FOR 1 WEEK, THEN 0.5 G BID FOR 2ND WEEK	5 G

Directions for reconstitution

ADD 6.5 ML STERILE WATER. RECONSTITUTED SOLUTION WILL CONTAIN 500 MG/1.0 ML. STORE IN REFRIGERATOR FOR NOT MORE THAN 14 DAYS.

$$\frac{1 g}{500 mg} = \frac{x}{1 ml}$$

$$\frac{1000 mg}{500 mg} = \frac{x}{1 ml}$$

$$500 x = 1000 \, ml$$

$$x = 2 \, ml$$

$$\frac{.5 g}{500 mg} = \frac{x}{1 ml}$$

$$\frac{500 mg}{500 mg} = \frac{x}{1 ml}$$

$$x = 1 \, ml$$

5.

Name: CANTRELL, ARTHUR	RM–BD: 268–A

Medication Order	**Available Medication**
PENICILLIN G 500,000 U IM Q4H	5,000,000 U

Directions for reconstitution

ADD 8 ML STERILE WATER. RECONSTITUTED
SOLUTION WILL CONTAIN 500,000 U/1.0 ML.

SOLUTION MAY BE KEPT IN REFRIGERATOR
FOR 1 WEEK WITHOUT LOSS OF POTENCY.

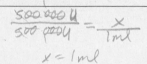

$$\frac{500,000\,U}{500,000\,U} = \frac{x}{1\,ml}$$

$$x = 1\,ml$$

6.

Name: LOPEZ, RAUL	RM–BD: 742–2

Medication Order	**Available Medication**
AMPICILLIN 500 MG IM Q6H	500 MG

Directions for reconstitution

ADD 1.7 ML STERILE WATER.
RECONSTITUTED SOLUTION WILL CONTAIN
250 MG/1.0 ML, AND MUST BE USED WITHIN
1 HOUR.

$$\frac{500\,mg}{250\,mg} = \frac{x}{1\,ml}$$

$$250x = 500\,ml$$

$$x = 2\,ml$$

7.

Name: GOLDBERG, MOLLIE	RM-BD: 107-A

Medication Order	Available Medication
TICARCILLIN DI- SODIUM 1 G IM TID	3 G

Directions for reconstitution

ADD 6 ML STERILE WATER. RECONSTITUTED
SOLUTION WILL CONTAIN 1 G/2.5 ML AND
IS STABLE FOR 24 HOURS AT ROOM
TEMPERATURE AND FOR 72 HOURS IF
REFRIGERATED.

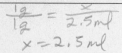

$$\frac{1g}{1g} = \frac{x}{2.5 ml}$$

$$x = 2.5 ml$$

Passing score is no more than *1* error.

On occasion, the directions for reconstitution may specify the amount of sterile water to add for various concentrations of medication.

For example:

> penicillin G–potassium
>
> 1,000,000 units

> Directions for reconstitution:
>
> Add 9.6 ml, 4.6 ml, or 3.6 ml sterile water to provide 100,000 U, 200,000 U, or 250,000 U/1.0 ml, respectively.

The above directions indicate that adding 9.6 ml sterile water will provide 100,000 units/1.0 ml, adding 4.6 ml sterile water will provide 200,000 units/1.0 ml, and adding 3.6 ml sterile water will provide a concentration of 250,000 units/1.0 ml.

One of the things you will have to determine is which concentration to use. For example, consider the following printout:

Name: JACKSON, GLORIA	RM–BD: 310–A

Medication Order	Available Medication
PENICILLIN G 200,000 U IM QID	1,000,000 U

Directions for reconstitution

ADD 9.6 ML, 4.6 ML, OR 3.6 ML TO
PROVIDE 100,000 U, 200,000 U, OR
250,000 U/1.0 ML, RESPECTIVELY.

1. Which concentration would you choose to prepare? *200,000 U/1ml*

2. How much sterile water would you add to the vial? *4.6ml*

3. How much solution would you give the patient? *1ml*

4. How would the medication be administered, and how often? *IM QID*

5. How would you relabel the vial? *200,000U/1.0ml*
   Time & date

Read the following label:

Penicillin G 5,000,000 U—add 23 ml, 18 ml, 8 ml, or 3 ml sterile water to provide 200,000 U, 250,000 U, 500,000 U, or 1,000,000 U/1.0 ml, respectively.

6. How much sterile water should be added to the vial to prepare each of the following concentrations?
   (a) 500,000 U/1.0 ml *8ml*
   (b) 1,000,000 U/1.0 ml *3ml*
   (c) 200,000 U/1.0 ml *23 ml*
   (d) 250,000 U/1.0 ml *18 ml*

7. The doctor's order reads "1,000,000 U penicillin G IM b.i.d." Which of the above concentrations would you select? *1,000,000U/1.0ml*

8. How much sterile water should you add for the concentration you need? *3ml*

9. How much solution should you give the patient? *1ml*

10. How often should the medication be administered? *bid*

11. How should you relabel the vial?
    1,000,000U/1.0ml time/date

Passing score is no more than *1* error.

Chapter 15

Intravenous Medications

Section 1 IV Rates for Adults

Many medications are given intravenously over a designated period of time. For instance, a doctor may order:

500 ml of glucose to be administered IV in 6 hours

The rate at which medication is given IV is measured in terms of *drops per minute.* Let's consider how to determine the number of *drops per minute* from the information provided in the doctor's order.

One of the factors that determines the number of drops per minute that should be given to the patient is the size of the drops. Some equipment delivers larger drops than other equipment. For example, one type of equipment delivers 10 drops per milliliter of liquid; another delivers 12 drops per milliliter; a third delivers 15 drops per milliliter.

The number of drops that the equipment delivers per milliliter of liquid is called the *drop factor.* In most cases, the *drop factor* is indicated on the equipment itself. Here's how the *drop factor* affects the number of drops per minute.

Example 1:

A patient is to be given a medication IV at the rate of 3 ml per minute. The equipment being used to administer the liquid delivers 15 drops per milliliter.

ml/minute × drops/ml = drops/minute

In this example, there are:

3 ml/minute
15 drops/ml

Therefore,

$$3 \text{ ml/minute} \times 15 \text{ drops/ml} = 45 \text{ drops/minute}$$

Example 2:

A patient is to be given 3 ml per minute IV using equipment that has a drop factor of 10 drops per milliliter.

In this example, there are:

$$3 \text{ ml/minute}$$
$$10 \text{ drops/ml}$$

Therefore,

$$3 \text{ ml/minute} \times 10 \text{ drops/ml} = 30 \text{ drops/minute.}$$

It is significant to note that in both Example 1 and Example 2, the patient is to receive 3 ml per minute IV. However, as a result of the variation in the *drop factor,* the patient in Example 1 should receive 45 drops per minute and the patient in Example 2 should receive 30 drops per minute.

Frequently, the nurse must calculate the number of drops per minute the patient should be given IV from the information that appears in the doctor's order. For example:

The doctor orders 600 ml of 5% glucose to be administered IV in 6 hours.

The nurse must determine the number of drops per minute the patient should receive so that at the end of 6 hours, he will have been given 600 ml.

In order to determine the *number of drops per minute,* the nurse must know the *drop factor* for the equipment being used to administer the medication. Keep in mind that the *drop factor* is the number of drops the equipment will deliver per milliliter of liquid. Assume that in this instance, the equipment will deliver 15 drops per milliliter of medication. Read the following step-by-step procedures carefully.

Step 1. *Determine the number of minutes the medication is to flow.*

Number of hours $\times$ 60 = Number of minutes

If the doctor ordered 600 ml in 6 hours, you must first convert 6 hours to minutes.

$$6 \text{ hours} \times 60 \text{ minutes/hour} = 360 \text{ minutes}$$

Step 2. *Determine the number of milliliters that the patient is to receive per minute.*

$$\frac{\text{Number of ml ordered}}{\substack{\text{Number of minutes the} \\ \text{medication is to flow}}} = \text{Number of ml/minute}$$

If the doctor ordered 600 ml IV in 360 minutes,

$$\frac{600 \text{ ml}}{360 \text{ min}} = \frac{10}{6} \text{ ml/min}$$

Step 3. *Determine the number of drops per minute to give the patient.*

$$\text{ml/min} \times \text{drop factor} = \text{drops/min}$$

If the ml/min is $\frac{10}{6}$ and the *drop factor* is 15 drops/ml,

$$\frac{10}{6} \text{ ml/min} \times 15 \text{ drops/ml} = 25 \text{ drops/min}$$

Step 4. *If necessary, round off the result to the nearest whole number.*

If the number of drops/min is not a whole number, round off to the closest whole number. 25.7 drops/min would be rounded off to 26 drops/min. 36.3 drops/min would be rounded off to 36 drops/min.

Let's try a few practice problems using these simple step-by-step procedures.

Answer the following questions.

1. The doctor ordered 1,500 ml of 10% glucose IV in 8 hours.

In order to determine the number of drops per minute, what must the nurse know about the equipment that will be used to administer the medication?

2. Determine the number of minutes the medication is to flow.

3. Determine the number of milliliters the patient is to receive per minute.

4. Determine the number of drops per minute. Assume that the drop factor is 10 drops/ml.

5. Round off the result.

The doctor ordered 1,000 ml of 10% glucose IV in 5 hours. What should be the rate of flow of the IV if the drop factor is 12?

6. Determine the number of minutes the medication is to flow.

7. Determine the number of milliliters that the patient is to receive per minute.

8. Determine the number of drops per minute.

Give 1,200 ml IV in 8 hours. The drop factor is 15.

9. Determine the number of minutes the medication is to flow.

10. Determine the number of milliliters that the patient is to receive per minute.

11. Determine the number of drops per minute.

12. Round off the result.

Passing score is no more than *1* error.

Now that you understand the steps involved in determining the *drops per minute,* let's consider a simple formula you may use.

$$\frac{\text{Number of ml ordered}}{\substack{\text{Number of min} \\ \text{medication is to flow}}} \times \text{Drop factor} = \substack{\text{Number of} \\ \text{drops/min}}$$

Let's consider an example using this formula.

The doctor ordered 500 ml of 10% glucose to be adminis-tered IV in 6 hours. If the equipment has a drop factor of 15, at what rate should the IV flow be adjusted?

Before using the formula, you must determine the *number of minutes the medication is to flow.*

In this case,

$$6 \text{ hours} \times 60 = 360 \text{ minutes}$$

Using the formula

$$\frac{\text{Number of ml ordered}}{\substack{\text{Number of min} \\ \text{medication is to flow}}} \times \text{Drop factor} = \text{Number of drops/min}$$

$$\frac{500 \text{ ml}}{360 \text{ min}} \times 15 = \text{Number of drops/min}$$

$$\frac{500}{360} \times 15 = \frac{7{,}500}{360} = 20.8 = 21 \text{ drops/min}$$

Let's try a few practice problems using this formula.

13. Give 800 ml IV in 4 hours. The drop factor is 12. Determine the number of drops per minute.

$$\frac{\text{No. of ml ordered}}{\substack{\text{No. of min} \\ \text{medication is to} \\ \text{flow}}} \times \text{Drop factor} = \text{No. drops/min}$$

14. Give 800 ml IV in 4 hours. The drop factor is 10. Determine the number of drops/min.

$$\frac{\text{No. of ml ordered}}{\substack{\text{No. of min the} \\ \text{medication is to flow}}} \times \text{Drop factor} = \text{No. drops/min}$$

In each of the following problems determine the number of drops per minute to give the patient when the drop factor is (a) 15, (b) 10, (c) 12.

1.

IV ORDER	
Name: KLASSER, BRIAN	**RM–BD:** 109–4
1,000 ML 5% GLUCOSE 10 HR	

2.

IV ORDER	
Name: ERICSON, ANDREW	**RM–BD:** 330–D
1,200 ML 5% D/W 8 HR	

3.

IV ORDER	
Name: BURDEN, EILEEN	**RM–BD:** 402–A
800 ML 5% GLUCOSE 4 HR	

4.

IV ORDER	
Name: CRUZ, MARIO	**RM–BD:** 874–3
1,250 ML 5% D/W 6 HR	

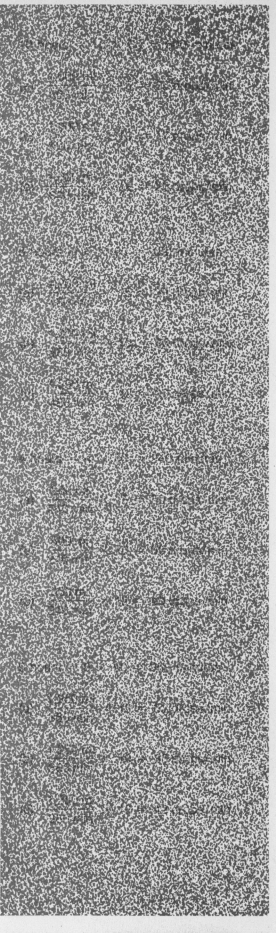

5.

IV ORDER	
Name: ALTER, GLADYS	**RM–BD:** 882–A
900 ML 10% GLUCOSE 4.5 HR	

6.

IV ORDER	
Name: BAXTER, MARLENE	**RM–BD:** 400–1
400 ML N/S 2 HR	

7.

IV ORDER	
Name: CARDEW, MAX	**RM–BD:** 708–2
500 ML 5% D/W 3 HR	

8.

IV ORDER	
Name: COX, OWEN	**RM–BD:** 1043–B
600 ML 10% GLUCOSE 2.5 HR	

Passing score is no more than *1* error.

Section 2 IV Deficit

Assume that a patient is supposed to receive 500 ml of medication over a 4-hour period. If the drop factor is 15, the rate of flow should be 31 drops per minute. However, during any period of time, an IV's rate of flow may vary according to the position of the patient's arm, the volume of IV left in the bottle, and the way the patient moves in bed.

In the above example, the patient should be receiving 125 ml per hour (500 ml per 4 hours). However, when a nurse checks the patient's IV, she may find that the patient has not received the required volume of medication. For example, suppose that at the end of the second hour, the patient has only received 200 ml instead of 250 ml. When this happens, the patient is said to have an IV deficit. This deficit should be made up by increasing the IV rate of flow. Here's the way to calculate the new flow rate.

Consider the following printout:

IV ORDER
Name: BREWER, MARION   **RM–BD:** 554–C
1,000 ML RINGER'S LACTATE 6 HR

1. If the drop factor is 15, what should be the rate of IV flow?

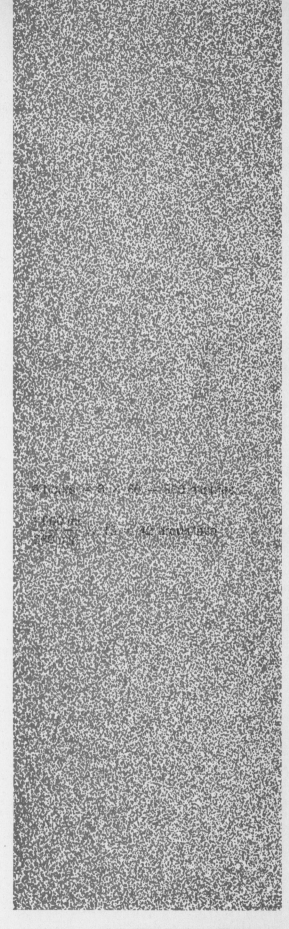

| | | | | Nursing Office
March, 1983

Date _March 24, 1983_ |
| | | | | |

IV Order Worksheet

IV #	Solution, Additives, Rate (K.O. 8°, etc.)	Time Started	Time Completed	Amount Left at End of Shift		
				0700	1500	2300
1	Room: _554-C_ Name: _Brewer, Marion_ 1,000 ML Ringer's Lactate 6 Hr	1100	1700	360		
2	Room: _190-A_ Name: _Orberg, Pamela_ 1,000 ML 5% D/W 6 HR 1,000 ML Ringer's Lactate 6 HR	0700 1300	1300 1900	700		
3	Room: _612-2_ Name: _Sanderson, Eileen_ 1500 ML 5% D/W 8 HR	1900	0300		800	
4	Room: _118-3_ Name: _Quigley, Marjorie_ 1,000 ML 5% D/W 8 HR 1,000 ML Ringer's Lactate 8 HR	0300 1100	1100 1900	600		

Figure 15-1. Sample IV order worksheet.

Now look at the following IV order worksheet for the same patient.

IV ORDER WORKSHEET

NAME: Brewer, Marion		RM–BD: 554–C			
	TIME START	TIME END	AMT LEFT AT END OF SHIFT		
			0700	1500	2300
1,000 ml Ringer's lactate 6 hr	1100	1700	360		

2. What time does the 0700 shift end?

3. At 1500, how long had the IV run?

4. At 1500, how much longer does the IV have to flow?

5. At 1500, how much IV fluid remains?

(Note: The amount under 0700 indicates the amount left at the *end* of the shift that began at 0700.)

6. What should be the new rate of IV flow (drop factor 15) for the remaining amount of IV fluid in the time left?

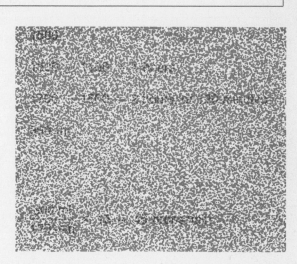

Consider the following:

IV ORDER WORKSHEET

NAME: Orberg, Pamela		RM–BD: 190–A			
	TIME START	TIME END	AMT LEFT AT END OF SHIFT		
			0700	1500	2300
1,000 ml 5% D/W 6 hr	0700	1300			
1,000 ml Ringer's lactate 6 hr	1300	1900	700		

Assuming a drop factor of 15, what will be the rate of flow of the first IV bottle?

7. What will be the original rate of flow of the second IV bottle?

8. How much IV fluid is left in the second bottle at 1500?

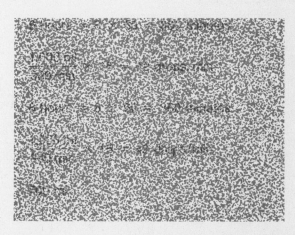

9. At 1500, how much time is left for the IV to run?

10. What will be the revised rate of IV flow?

For each of the following problems, calculate the original rate of IV flow and the revised rate of flow.

1.

IV ORDER WORKSHEET

NAME: Sunderson, Eileen		RM–BD: 612–2			
				AMT LEFT AT END OF SHIFT	
	TIME START	TIME END	0700	1500	2300
1,500 ml 5% D/W 8 hr	1900	0300		800	

(Assume a drop factor of 15.)

2.

IV ORDER WORKSHEET

NAME: Quigley, Marjorie		RM–BD: 118–3			
				AMT LEFT AT END OF SHIFT	
	TIME START	TIME END	0700	1500	2300
1,000 ml 5% D/W 8 hr	0300	1100			
1,000 ml Ringer's lactate 8 hr	1100	1900	600		

(Assume a drop factor of 10.)

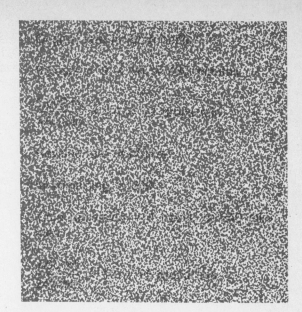

3.

IV ORDER WORKSHEET

NAME: Hokawa, Sei	RM–BD: 664–1				
				AMT LEFT AT END OF SHIFT	
	TIME START	TIME END	0700	1500	2300
2,000 ml 5% D/W 12 hr	2300	1100			750

(Assume a drop factor of 10.)

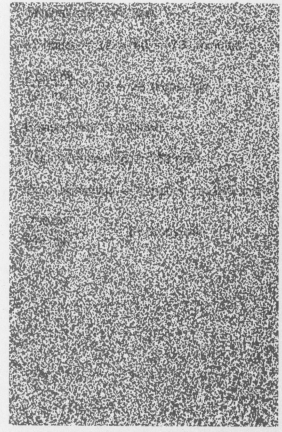

Passing score is no more than *1* error.

Section 3   IV Rates for Infants

When an IV medication is given to an adult, the rate of flow is measured in terms of *drops per minute*. Infants are given much smaller dosages of medications, and therefore, when an infant is given an intravenous infusion, the rate of flow is measured in terms of *microdrops per minute*. A great deal of the equipment that is used to give intravenous infusions to an infant provides 60 microdrops per milliliter. The same formula is used to determine the *number of microdrops per minute to give an infant.*

$$\frac{\text{No. of ml ordered}}{\substack{\text{No. of min the}\\ \text{medication is to flow}}} \times \substack{\text{Drop}\\ \text{factor}} = \substack{\text{No.}\\ \text{microdrops/min}}$$

Let's consider an example using this formula. The patient is an infant and the drop factor is 60 microdrops/ml.

IV ORDER
Name: GORDON, ROSA   **RM–BD:** 114–3
100 ML 10% GLUCOSE 4 HR

4 hours $= 4 \times 60 = 240$ minutes

$$\frac{100 \text{ ml}}{240 \text{ min}} \times 60 \text{ microdrops/ml} = 25 \text{ microdrops/min}$$

In each of the following problems determine the number of microdrops per minute to give an infant when the drop factor is 60 microdrops/ml.*

1.

IV ORDER
Name: KARLEY, SANDRA   **RM–BD:** 109–C
120 ML PHYSIOLOGIC SALINE 6 HR

* Throughout the book, decimals are rounded to whole numbers. Whenever a result is expressed as .5 or .50, round to the nearest even number. Thus, 12.5 is rounded to 12, while 13.5 is rounded to 14.

2.

IV ORDER
Name: PRENTICE, IAN   **RM–BD:** 204–1
60 ML RINGER'S LACTATE 3 HR

3.

IV ORDER
Name: SWANE, BRENDA   **RM–BD:** 330–A
100 ML 5% GLUCOSE 8 HR

4.

IV ORDER
Name: THOMPSON, JEANNE   **RM–BD:** 229–2
150 ML 5% D/W 8 HR

5.

IV ORDER
Name: HILKER, ANNA   **RM–BD:** 340–2
80 ML 10% GLUCOSE 2.5 HR

Passing score is no more than *1* error.

Section 4   Time of Running for IV Medications

When the doctor orders an intravenous medication, he may specify the rate at which it is to be administered. Consider the following order.

IV ORDER
Name: HUTTNER, ALEXANDER   **RM–BD:** 300–2
1,200 ML 0.9% SALINE 50 DROPS/MIN

In such cases, the nurse must calculate the length of time the IV is to run. Please read the following step-by-step procedures carefully.

Step 1. *Determine the total number of drops ordered.*

$$\genfrac{}{}{0pt}{}{\text{Number of ml}}{\text{ordered}} \times \genfrac{}{}{0pt}{}{\text{Drop}}{\text{factor}} = \text{Total number of drops}$$

If the doctor ordered 1,200 ml and the drop factor is 15 drops/ml,

$$1{,}200 \text{ ml} \times 15 \text{ drops/ml} = 18{,}000 \text{ drops}$$

Step 2. *Determine the number of minutes the medication is to flow.*

$$\frac{\text{Total number of drops}}{\text{Number of drops/min}} = \genfrac{}{}{0pt}{}{\text{Number of min medication}}{\text{is to flow}}$$

If the patient receives 18,000 drops at the rate of 50 drops/min,

$$\frac{18{,}000 \text{ drops}}{50 \text{ drops/min}} = 360 \text{ min}$$

Step 3. *Convert minutes to hours and minutes.*

$$\frac{360 \text{ min}}{60} = 6 \text{ hours}$$

Let's try a practice problem.

IV ORDER
Name: CHUNG, HAZEL   **RM–BD:** 207–A
900 ML 5% D/W   40 DROPS/MIN

(Assume a drop factor of 10.)

1. Determine the total number of drops ordered.

2. Determine the number of minutes the medication is to flow.

3. Convert minutes to hours and minutes.

IV ORDER

Name: QUARREN, RAFAEL	**RM–BD:** 337–1

80 ML RINGER'S LACTATE 20 MICRODROPS/MIN

(Assume a drop factor of 60.)

4. Determine the total number of microdrops ordered.

5. Determine the number of minutes the medication is to flow.

6. Convert minutes to hours.

Now that you understand the steps involved in determining the length of time the IV is to run, let's consider a formula you may use.

$$\frac{\text{Number of ml ordered}}{\substack{\text{Number of min the} \\ \text{medication is to run}}} \times \substack{\text{Drop} \\ \text{factor}} = \substack{\text{No.} \\ \text{drops/min}}$$

Consider an example using this formula.

IV ORDER

Name: STONE, MELVIN	**RM–BD:** 1210–4

1,200 ML NORMAL SALINE 50 DROPS/MIN

How long should the IV run? Assume a drop factor of 15.

Using the formula,

$$\frac{\text{Number of ml ordered}}{\substack{\text{Number of min the} \\ \text{medication is to run}}} \times \text{Drop factor} = \text{No. drops/min}$$

$$\frac{1{,}200 \text{ ml}}{X} \times 15 = 50 \text{ drops/min}$$

where X is the number of minutes the medication is to flow.

Step 1.   *Multiply the number of milliliters ordered by the drop factor to determine the total number of drops ordered.*

$$1{,}200 \text{ ml} \times 15 \text{ drops/ml} = 18{,}000 \text{ drops}$$

Step 2.   *Substitute the result in the formula.*

$$\frac{18{,}000 \text{ drops}}{X} = 50 \text{ drops/min}$$

Step 3.   *Cross-multiply.*

$$50X = 18{,}000$$

$$X = \frac{18{,}000}{50} = 360 \text{ min}$$

Step 4.   *Convert minutes to hours.*

$$\frac{360 \text{ min}}{60} = 6 \text{ hours}$$

Let's try another practice problem using this formula and the step-by-step procedure.

IV ORDER
Name: SWENSEN, OLAF   **RM–BD:** 403–B
1,000 ML 10% GLUCOSE   35 DROPS/MIN

(Assume a drop factor of 10.)

7.   Substitute the appropriate values in the following formula.

$$\frac{\text{Number of ml ordered}}{\substack{\text{Number of min the} \\ \text{medication is to flow}}} \times \substack{\text{Drop} \\ \text{factor}} = \text{No. drops/min}$$

8. Multiply the number of milliliters ordered by the drop factor to determine the total number of drops ordered. Substitute the result in the formula.

9. Cross-multiply.

10. Convert minutes to hours.

Passing score is no more than *1* error.

In each of the following problems determine the approximate time that the IV medication should run.

1.

IV ORDER	
Name: COOKE, MYLES	**RM–BD:** 107-2
900 ML 5% D/W 40 DROPS/MIN	

(The drop factor is 15 drops/ml.)

2.

IV ORDER	
Name: BRANDER, JACKSON	**RM–BD:** 235-3
80 ML 10% GLUCOSE 20 MICRODROPS/MIN	

(The drop factor is 60 microdrops/ml.)

3.

IV ORDER	
Name: MARTINEZ, MIGUEL	**RM–BD:** 382-C
60 ML 5% D/W 24 MICRODROPS/MIN	

(The drop factor is 60 microdrops/ml.)

$\frac{60 \text{ ml}}{X} \times 60 = 24$ microdrops/min

$60 \times 60 = 3{,}600$

$\frac{3{,}600}{X} = 24$

$24X = 3{,}600$

$X = 150$ min, or $2\frac{1}{2}$ hours

4.

IV ORDER	
Name: DRINON, MARCUS	**RM–BD:** 500-3
1,500 ML RINGER'S LACTATE 50 DROPS/MIN	

(The drop factor is 10 drops/ml.)

$\frac{1{,}500 \text{ ml}}{X} \times 10 = 50$ drops/min

$1{,}500 \times 10 = 15{,}000$

$\frac{15{,}000 \text{ drops}}{X} = 50$ drops/min

$50X = 15{,}000$

$X = 300$ min, or 5 hours

5.

IV ORDER	
Name: COHEN, BRANDON	**RM–BD:** 405-1
90 ML 5% D/W 30 MICRODROPS/MIN	

(The drop factor is 60 microdrops/ml.)

$\frac{90 \text{ ml}}{X} \times 60 = 30$ microdrops/min

$90 \times 60 = 5{,}400$ microdrops

$\frac{5{,}400 \text{ microdrops}}{X} = 30$ microdrops/min

$30X = 5{,}400$

$X = 180$ min, or 3 hours

6.

IV ORDER	
Name: HERMAN, GENE	**RM–BD:** 412-1
750 ML PHYSIOLOGIC SALINE 40 DROPS/MIN	

(The drop factor is 12 drops/ml.)

$\frac{750 \text{ ml}}{X} \times 12 = 40$ drops/min

$750 \text{ ml} \times 12 = 9{,}000$ drops

$\frac{9{,}000 \text{ drops}}{X} = 40$ drops/min

$40X = 9{,}000$

$X = 225$ min, or $3\frac{3}{4}$ hours

7.

IV ORDER	
Name: DUNCAN, NANCY	**RM–BD:** 205–3
100 ML 10% GLUCOSE 25 MICRODROPS/MIN	

(The drop factor is 60 microdrops/ml.)

$$\frac{100 \text{ ml}}{X} \times 60 = 25 \text{ microdrops/min}$$

$100 \text{ ml} \times 60 = 6{,}000$ microdrops

$$\frac{6{,}000 \text{ microdrops}}{X} = 25 \text{ microdrops/min}$$

$25X = 6{,}000$

$X = 240$ min, or 4 hours

8.

IV ORDER	
Name: TAYLOR, THELMA	**RM–BD:** 690–A
1,000 ML RINGER'S LACTATE 40 DROPS/MIN	

(The drop factor is 15.)

$$\frac{1{,}000 \text{ ml}}{X} \times 15 = 40 \text{ drops/min}$$

$1{,}000 \text{ ml} \times 15 = 15{,}000$ drops

$$\frac{15{,}000 \text{ drops}}{X} = 40 \text{ drops/min}$$

$40X = 15{,}000$

$X = 375$ min, or $6\frac{1}{4}$ hours

9.

IV ORDER	
Name: PAULSON, CINDY	**RM–BD:** 759–4
125 ML 10% GLUCOSE 50 MICRODROPS/MIN	

(The drop factor is 60.)

$$\frac{125 \text{ ml}}{X} \times 60 = 50 \text{ microdrops/min}$$

$125 \text{ ml} \times 60 = 7{,}500$ microdrops

$$\frac{7{,}500 \text{ microdrops}}{X} = 50 \text{ microdrops/min}$$

$50X = 7{,}500$

$X = 150$ min, or $2\frac{1}{2}$ hours

10.

IV ORDER
Name: FROMER, PAUL **RM–BD:** 447–3
750 ML 10% GLUCOSE 60 DROPS/MIN

(The drop factor is 10.)

Passing score is no more than *2* errors.

Section 5 Time of Running for IV Medications (cont.)

Consider the following printout:

IV ORDER
Name: SINDRON, TESI **RM–BD:** 602–4
1,000 ML 5% D/W 200 ML/HR

In previous examples, the doctor ordered the IV to be given at the rate of a certain number of drops per minute. In this example the doctor has ordered the IV to be administered at a given number of milliliters per hour.

To determine the length of time that the IV will run, we use the following formula:

$$\frac{\textbf{Number of ml ordered}}{\textbf{Number of ml/hour}} = \textbf{Number of hours}$$

In this example, $\dfrac{1,000 \text{ ml}}{200 \text{ ml/hr}} = 5$ hours

If the drop factor is 15, at what rate should the IV flow? Recall the formula:

$$\frac{\text{Number of ml ordered}}{\substack{\text{Number of min} \\ \text{medication is to flow}}} \times \frac{\text{Drop}}{\text{factor}} = \frac{\text{Number of}}{\text{drops/min}}$$

1. How many ml were ordered?

2. How many minutes should the IV flow?

3. What should be the rate of IV flow?

For each of the following printouts, calculate the number of hours the IV is to flow and also the rate of flow, assuming a drop factor of 15.

1.

IV ORDER	
Name: TROUT, BRAD	**RM–BD:** 107–2
1,200 ML N/S 100 ML/HR	

2.

IV ORDER	
Name: HOOK, MELANIE	**RM–BD:** 208–C
750 ML 5% D/W 125 ML/HR	

3.

IV ORDER	
Name: TEMPLETON, OSCAR	**RM–BD:** 330–A
200 ML 5% D/W 50 ML/HR	

4.

IV ORDER	
Name: ZENDLER, BRUNO	**RM–BD:** 117–2
2,000 ML 5% D/W 125 ML/HR	

Passing score is no more than *1* error.

Chapter 16

Piggyback IV's

A doctor may order an IV medication to run piggyback (IVPB) with IV fluids. The order might read:

2,000 ml 5% D/W, 24 hr, + 1 g Keflin IVPB q.6h.

If the piggyback is prepared by the pharmacy, the computer printout might be:

IV ORDER
Name: MASON, STACEY   **RM–BD:** 904–A
2,000 ML 5% D/W   24 HR

Name: MASON, STACEY		**RM–BD:** 904–A
Medication Order	**Time**	**Available Medication**
KEFLIN 1 G IVPB Q6H	1 HR	1 G KEFLIN/100 ML 5% D/W

If the piggyback is prepared by the nurse on the floor, the computer printout might be:

IV ORDER	
Name: MASON, STACEY	**RM–BD:** 904–A
2,000 ML 5% D/W 24 HR	

Name: MASON, STACEY		**RM–BD:** 904–A
Medication Order	**Time**	**Available Medication**
KEFLIN 1 G IVPB Q6H	1 HR	1 G
Directions		
DISSOLVE IN 100 ML 5% D/W.		

Piggyback IV's are usually dissolved in either 50 ml or 100 ml of IV solution, the amount being specified in the directions, or package inserts.

When there is a piggyback medication, it is necessary to calculate the number of drops per minute both during the piggyback as well as between piggybacks.

As you have already learned, the following formula may be used:

$$\frac{\text{Number of ml ordered}}{\substack{\text{Number of min} \\ \text{medication is to flow}}} \times \substack{\textbf{Drop} \\ \textbf{factor}} = \substack{\textbf{Number of} \\ \textbf{drops/min}}$$

Read the following example carefully.

IV ORDER	
Name: BAXTER, MARILYN	**RM–BD:** 448–2
1,800 ML 5% D/W 24 HR	

Name: BAXTER, MARILYN		**RM–BD:** 448–2
Medication Order	**Time**	**Available Medication**
KEFLIN 500 MG IVPB Q4H	1 HR	500 MG/50 ML 5% D/W

Assume that you have to determine the number of drops of Keflin to administer per minute. According to the above order, the Keflin is dissolved in 50 ml 5% D/W and is to run for 1 hour. Try to answer the following questions, assuming a drop factor of 15.

1. Using the equation, determine the number of drops of Keflin solution to administer per minute.

In order to determine the number of drops per minute of IV fluid to administer between piggybacks, the nurse must first calculate the volume of IV fluid that should be given per hour. Read the following step-by-step procedures carefully.

Step 1. *Determine the number of times the piggyback medication is to be administered.*

In the above order, the IV is to run 24 hours. The piggyback medication is administered every 4 hours. Therefore, the piggyback medication will be given 6 times.

Step 2. *Determine the total volume of piggyback medication.*

The patient is to receive 50 ml of the piggyback medication each time it is to run. Therefore, 6 times × 50 ml per time = 300 ml.

Step 3. *Subtract the total volume of the piggyback medication from the total volume of IV fluids to be administered in order to determine the volume of IV fluids to be given between piggybacks.*

$$\text{Total volume of IV fluids} - \text{Total volume of piggybacks} = \text{Total volume to administer between piggybacks}$$

$$1{,}800 - 300 = 1{,}500 \text{ ml}$$

Step 4. *Determine the total time the piggyback medication is to run.*

The piggyback medication is to be given 6 times and run for 1 hour each time. Therefore, the piggyback medication will be administered for 6 hours.

Step 5. *Determine the total time between piggybacks by subtracting the piggyback time from the total time the IV is to flow.*

$$\text{Total time the IV is to flow} - \text{Total time for all piggybacks} = \text{Total time between piggybacks}$$

The IV is to flow for 24 hours; the piggyback is to flow for 6 hours. Therefore, the IV will flow for 18 hours between piggybacks.

Step 6. *Determine the number of drops per minute to adminis-ter between piggybacks using the following formula:*

$$\frac{\text{Number of ml ordered}}{\substack{\text{Number of min} \\ \text{medication is to flow}}} \times \text{Drop factor} = \text{Number of drops/min}$$

In the case of the order being considered,

$$\substack{\text{The number of ml to administer} \\ \text{between piggybacks}} = 1{,}500 \text{ ml}$$

The IV fluid is to flow for 18 hours between piggybacks. 18 hours × 60 minutes = 1,080 minutes.

The drop factor = 15

Therefore,

$$\frac{1{,}500 \text{ ml}}{1{,}080 \text{ min}} \times 15 = 21 \frac{\text{drops}}{\text{min}}$$

Let us consider another example.

IV ORDER		
Name: MOELLER, HANS		**RM–BD:** 501–1
2,500 ML 5% D/W 24 HR		

Name: MOELLER, HANS		**RM–BD:** 501–1
Medication Order	**Time**	**Available Medication**
AMPICILLIN 500 MG IVPB Q4H	30 MIN	500 MG
Directions		
DISSOLVE IN 50 ML 5% D/W.		

Assume that the medication has been dissolved in 50 ml 5% D/W and also that the drop factor is 10.

Answer the following questions.

2. Using the formula, determine the number of drops per minute to administer for the piggyback medication.

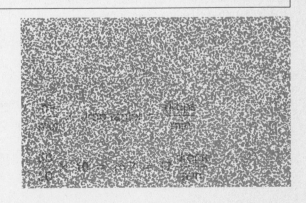

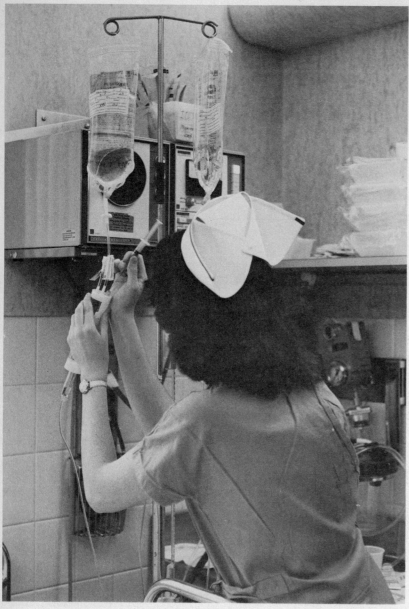

Figure 16-1. IV piggyback. (*Courtesy of School of Nursing, St. Francis Hospital, Evanston, Ill.*)

Assume that you need to determine the number of drops per minute of IV fluid to administer between piggybacks. In order to make the calculation, you must first determine the total volume of the piggyback medication. Try to answer the following step-by-step questions.

3. How many times is the piggyback medication to be administered?

4. Determine the total volume of piggyback medication.

5. Determine the total volume of IV fluid to be administered between piggybacks.

Total volume of IV fluids	−	Total volume of piggybacks	=	Total volume to administer between piggybacks

6. Determine the total time the piggyback medication is to run.

7. Determine the total time between piggybacks.

Total time the IV is to flow	−	Total time for all piggybacks	=	Total time between piggybacks

8. Determine the number of drops to administer between piggybacks.

$$\frac{\text{Number of ml ordered}}{\text{Number of min medication is to flow}} \times \frac{\text{Drop}}{\text{factor}} = \frac{\text{Number of}}{\text{drops/min}}$$

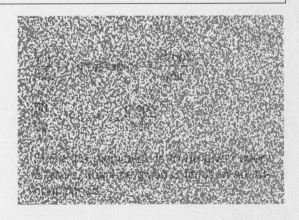

Let's consider another example.

IV ORDER		
Name: SAX, BRIAN		**RM–BD:** 207–3
2,000 ML NORMAL SALINE 18 HR		

Name: SAX, BRIAN		**RM–BD:** 207–3
Medication Order	**Time**	**Available Medication**
CHLORAMPHENICOL 500 MG IVPB Q6H	1 HR	500 MG/50 ML NORMAL SALINE

(Assume a drop factor of 15.)

9. Determine the number of drops per minute for the piggyback medication.

10. Determine the number of times the piggyback medication is to be administered.

11. Determine the total volume of all piggybacks.

12. Determine the total volume to be administered between piggybacks.

13. Determine the total time the IV is to flow between piggybacks.

14. Determine the drops per minute that should be administered between piggybacks.

IV ORDER	
Name: PORTER, ARNOLD	**RM–BD:** 108–3
1,500 ML NORMAL SALINE 24 HR	

Name: PORTER, ARNOLD		RM–BD: 108–3
Medication Order	**Time**	**Available Medication**
GENTAMICIN 80 MG IVPB Q6H	30 MIN	80 MG/2 ML
Directions		
DISSOLVE IN 100 ML NORMAL SALINE.		

Recall the formula:

$$\frac{\text{Desired amount}}{\text{Available amount}} = \frac{\text{How much we are going to use}}{\text{How much we have on hand}}$$

15. Calculate how much of the medication we are going to use.

16. According to the directions, what should be done with the 2 ml of solution?

The total volume of the piggyback will be 102 ml (100 ml + 2 ml). However, for all practical purposes, the piggyback is assumed to contain 100 ml.

17. Determine the number of drops per minute for the piggyback medication.

18. Determine the number of times the piggyback is to be administered.

19. Determine the total volume of all piggybacks.

20. Determine the total volume to be administered between piggybacks.

21. Determine the total time the IV is to flow between piggybacks.

22. Determine the drops per minute that should be administered between piggybacks.

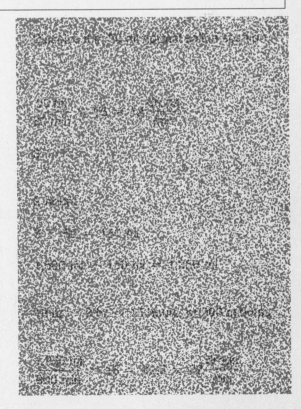

IV ORDER		
Name: STONE, BERNARD		**RM–BD:** 385–4
1,500 ML NORMAL SALINE 18 HR		

Name: STONE, BERNARD		**RM–BD:** 385–4
Medication Order	**Time**	**Available Medication**
AMPICILLIN 1 G IVPB Q6H	1 HR	1 G
Directions		
DISSOLVE IN 50 ML NORMAL SALINE.		

23. What should be done with the 1 g of ampicillin?

Assume that the total volume of the piggyback is 50 ml.

24. Determine the rate of flow of the piggyback. The drop factor is 15.

25. Determine the number of times the piggyback is to be administered.

26. Determine the total time for all piggybacks.

27. Determine the total volume of all piggybacks.

28. Determine the total volume to be administered between piggybacks.

29. Determine the total time the IV is to flow between piggybacks.

30. Determine the drops per minute that should be administered between piggybacks.

IV ORDER	
Name: ZENO, MARK	**RM–BD:** 763–D
3,000 ML 5% D/W 24 HR	

Name: ZENO, MARK		**RM–BD:** 763–D
Medication Order	**Time**	**Available Medication**
KEFLIN 1 G IVPB Q6H	30 MIN	1 G
Directions		
DISSOLVE IN 100 ML 5% D/W.		

(The drop factor is 15.)

31. Determine the flow rate of the piggyback.

32. Determine the flow rate between piggybacks.

Passing score is no more than *2* errors.

IV Piggybacks from Powdered Medications

Let's consider how to determine the number of drops per minute to administer when the piggyback is from a powdered medication. Consider the following order:

IV ORDER

Name: MARTIN, SARAH   **RM–BD:** 282–1

2,000 ML NORMAL SALINE   24 HR

Name: MARTIN, SARAH   **RM–BD:** 282–1

Medication Order	Time	Available Medication
AMPICILLIN 500 MG IVPB Q6H	1 HR	1 G

Directions for Reconstitution

INJECT 3.5 ML STERILE DILUENT. RECONSTITUTED SOLUTION WILL CONTAIN
250 MG/1 ML.

Directions for Piggyback

DISSOLVE IN 50 ML NORMAL SALINE.

When the medication is from a powder, the first thing you may have to determine is the volume of solution that is going to be administered. As you may recall, the following equation is used:

$$\frac{\text{Desired amount}}{\text{Available amount}} = \frac{\text{How much we are going to use}}{\text{How much we have on hand}}$$

Try to answer the following questions.

1. The label indicates that when 3.5 ml sterile diluent is added to the contents of the vial, the strength of the reconstituted solution will be 250 mg/1 ml. What is the available amount?

2. How much do we have on hand?

3. From the medication order, what is the desired amount?

4. Using the equation, calculate the volume we are going to use.

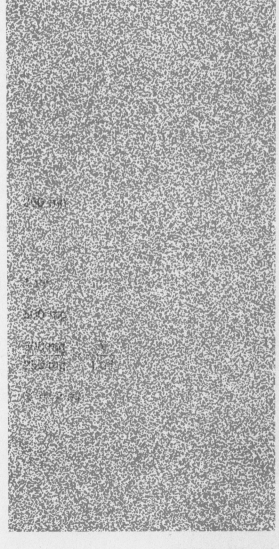

The order indicates that the medication is to be dissolved in 50 ml normal saline. Therefore, after the 3.5 ml diluent is injected into the vial, 2 ml of reconstituted ampicillin should be added to 50 ml of normal saline so that it can be administered IV as a piggyback.

As soon as you have determined the volume of piggyback medication, you can determine the number of drops per minute to administer both during the piggyback and between piggybacks.

In this example, 2 ml of reconstituted ampicillin is to be added to 50 ml of normal saline. Therefore, the total volume of the piggyback is really 52 ml. However, for practical purposes, the total volume of the piggyback is assumed to be 50 ml.

In some cases, the reconstituted medication is added to 100 ml of saline solution so that it can be administered as a piggyback. In that case, the volume of the piggyback is considered to be 100 ml.

5. What is the volume of ampicillin that must be administered during each piggyback?

6. If the drop factor is 10, how many drops per minute should be given during the piggyback?

7. The order indicates that the piggyback is to be administered q.6h. How many times will the piggyback be administered during a 24-hour period?

8. Determine the total volume of medication that is administered for all piggybacks. (Keep in mind that for practical purposes, 50 ml is administered per piggyback.)

9. The patient is to be given 2,000 ml during a 24-hour period. Determine the total volume that is to be administered between piggybacks.

10. Determine the total time the IV is to flow between piggybacks.

11. Determine the drops per minute that should be administered between piggybacks.

Let's try another example. Read the following order:

<table>
<tr><td colspan="2" align="center">**IV ORDER**</td></tr>
<tr><td>**Name:** CHELTON, HERMAN</td><td>**RM–BD:** 665–C</td></tr>
<tr><td colspan="2">1,500 ML 5% D/W 16 HR</td></tr>
</table>

Name: CHELTON, HERMAN		**RM–BD:** 665–C
Medication Order	**Time**	**Available Medication**
1,500,000 U PENICILLIN IVPB Q4H	30 MIN	5,000,000 U

Directions for Reconstitution

INJECT 8.2 ML STERILE DILUENT. RECONSTITUTED SOLUTION WILL CONTAIN 500,000 U/1 ML.

Directions for Piggyback

DISSOLVE IN 100 ML 5% D/W.

Try to answer the following questions.

12. From the medication order, what is the desired amount of penicillin?

13. From the reconstituted solution, what is the available amount?

14. How much reconstituted solution do we have on hand?

15. At this point, do you know how much of the reconstituted solution we are going to use?

16. Using the appropriate equation, determine how much we are going to use.

17. What should this 3 ml of reconstituted penicillin be dissolved in?

18. For practical purposes, what is the volume of the piggyback?

19. Determine the number of drops per minute for the piggyback. Assume a drop factor of 15.

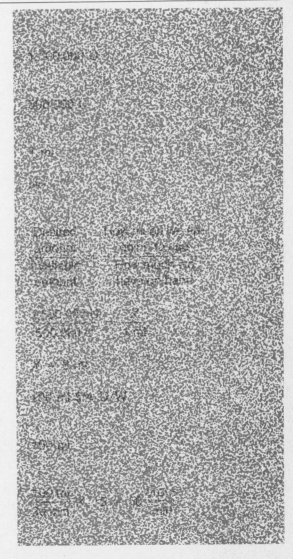

20. How many times will the piggyback be administered during a 16-hour period?

21. Determine the total volume of medication that is administered for all piggybacks. (Keep in mind that for practical purposes, 100 ml is administered per piggyback.)

22. Determine the total volume of the IV fluids that is to flow between piggybacks.

23. Determine the total time the IV is to flow between piggybacks.

24. Determine the drops per minute that should be administered between piggybacks.

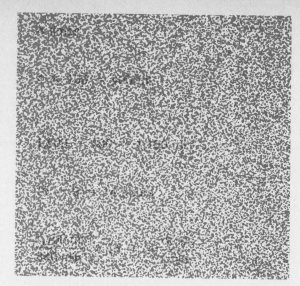

Consider the following order:

IV ORDER	
Name: BREADWAY, MAX	**RM–BD:** 603–A
1,800 ML NORMAL SALINE 18 HR	

Name: BREADWAY, MAX		**RM–BD:** 603–A
Medication Order	**Time**	**Available Medication**
GENTAMICIN 100 MG IVPB Q6H	1 HR	80 MG/2 ML
Directions		
DISSOLVE IN 50 ML NORMAL SALINE.		

25. Use the formula

$$\frac{\text{Desired amount}}{\text{Available amount}} = \frac{\text{How much we are going to use}}{\text{How much we have on hand}}$$

to determine how much solution to use for each piggyback.

26. What should be done with the 2.5 ml of gentamicin solution?

27. What volume will each piggyback have, on a practical basis?

28. Determine the number of drops per minute that should be administered for the piggybacks. Assume a drop factor of 15.

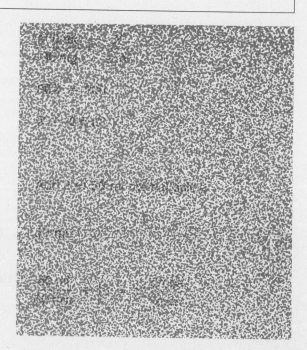

29. Determine the number of drops per minute to administer between the piggybacks.

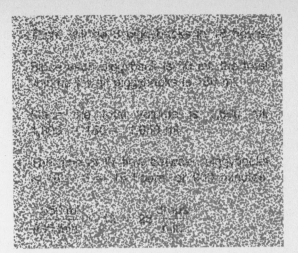

Consider the following order:

IV ORDER
Name: BURTON, JOSEPH   **RM–BD:** 338–3
1,500 ML 5% D/W   12 HR

Name: BURTON, JOSEPH		**RM–BD:** 338–3
Medication Order	**Time**	**Available Medication**
PENICILLIN G 1,000,000 U IVPB Q4H	1 HR	5,000,000 U
Directions		
INJECT 18.2 ML STERILE DILUENT. RECONSTITUTED SOLUTION WILL CONTAIN 250,000 U/1 ML.		
Directions for Piggyback		
DISSOLVE IN 50 ML 5% D/W.		

30. Determine the amount of reconstituted solution to use for each piggyback.

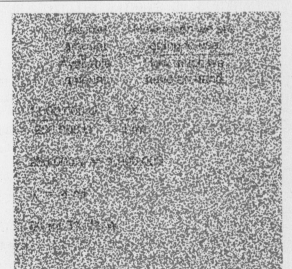

31. The 4 ml of reconstituted penicillin solution is dissolved in how much liquid?

32. Determine the number of drops per minute that should be administered for the piggybacks. The drop factor is 15.

33. Determine the number of drops per minute to give between piggybacks.

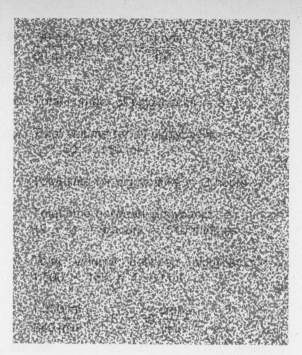

Consider the following order:

IV ORDER
Name: MENDELSON, MARTIN   **RM–BD:** 605-2
2,500 ML NORMAL SALINE 24 HR

Name: MENDELSON, MARTIN		**RM–BD:** 605-2
Medication Order	**Time**	**Available Medication**
KEFLIN 500 MG IVPB Q6H	30 MIN	1 G

Directions for Reconstitution

INJECT 5 ML STERILE DILUENT. RECONSTITUTED SOLUTION WILL CONTAIN 200 MG/1 ML.

Directions for Piggyback

DISSOLVE IN 100 ML NORMAL SALINE.

34. Determine the amount of reconstituted solution to use for each piggyback.

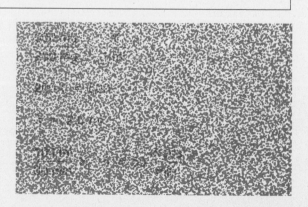

35. Determine the number of drops per minute to administer per piggyback. The drop factor is 15.

36. Determine the number of drops per minute to administer between piggybacks.

Passing score is no more than *2* errors.

Chapter 17

Calories from IV Medications

The body metabolizes glucose to produce energy. This is true whether the glucose is taken orally, is produced from other carbohydrates, or is administered intravenously. It has been established that the body produces 4 Cal of heat energy whenever it metabolizes 1 g of glucose. Therefore, the total number of Calories is determined by the following formula:

No. of g of glucose $\times$ 4 Cal/g = Total Cal

For example, assume that the body metabolizes 2 g of glucose. How many Calories did the body produce?

$$2 \text{ g} \times 4 \text{ Cal/g} = 8 \text{ Cal}$$

It should be noted that the body will produce 4 Cal of heat energy for every gram of glucose no matter how the body received that glucose. Another point to remember is that glucose is a carbohydrate. The body produces 4 Cal of heat energy upon the metabolism of 1 g of any carbohydrate.

The nurse may be called upon to determine the number of Calories of heat energy the body will produce as a result of being given a certain amount of glucose IV.

Consider the following example:

A patient is given 500 ml of 10% glucose solution intravenously. How many Calories did the patient receive?

Observe that in this example the patient is given 500 ml IV. Since 1 ml weighs 1 g, 500 ml weighs 500 g. However, only 10% of this weight is glucose. Therefore, 10% of 500 g = 50 g of glucose. For every gram of glucose that the body metabolizes, the body produces 4 Cal. Therefore,

$$50 \text{ g} \times 4 \text{ Cal/g} = 200 \text{ Cal}$$

Let's consider another example.

An infant receives 100 ml of 5% glucose IV. How many Calories were administered to the infant?

Step 1. *Determine the number of grams of glucose being administered.*

Since 1 ml weighs 1 g, 100 ml weighs 100 g

5% of 100 g = 5 g

Step 2. *Determine the number of Calories.*

5 g × 4 Cal/g = 20 Cal

When the body metabolizes protein and protein hydrolysate, again 4 Cal are produced for every gram metabolized. Let's consider an example.

A patient receives 500 ml of 5% protein hydrolysate IV. How many Calories did the patient receive?

Step 1. *Determine the number of grams being administered.*

500 ml = 500 g

5% of 500 g = 25 g protein

Step 2. *Determine the number of Calories.*

Note that each gram of protein hydrolysate yields 4 Cal.

25 g × 4 Cal/g = 100 Cal

Let's consider a few practice problems.

An infant is given 120 ml of 5% glucose IV. How many Calories were administered?

1. Determine the number of grams of glucose.

2. Determine the number of Calories.

A patient is given 1,000 ml of 10% glucose IV in 6 hours. How many Calories were administered?

3. Determine the number of grams of glucose.

4. Determine the number of Calories.

Consider the following example.

A patient is given 1 Liter of solution IV. The solution contains 800 ml of 5% protein hydrolysate, 150 ml of 50% glucose, and 50 ml of saline solution. How many Calories did the patient receive?

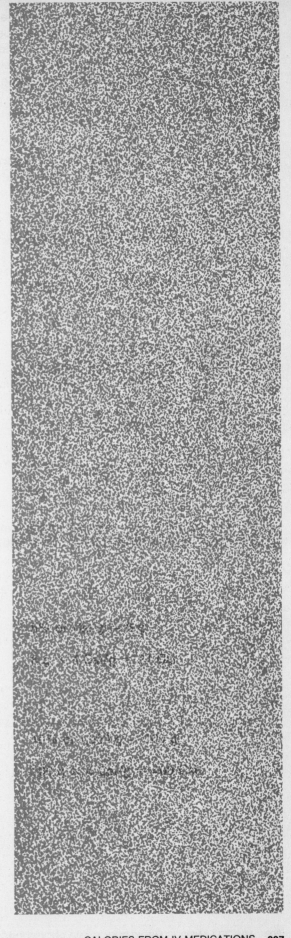

Since the body will not produce any Calories from saline solution, it has no effect upon the total number of Calories given. In this case the total number of Calories is equal to the number of Calories in the 800 ml of protein hydrolysate plus the Calories in the 150 ml of 50% glucose.

The following step-by-step procedures are used to determine the total number of Calories.

Step 1. *Determine the number of grams of protein hydrolysate.*

$$5\% \text{ of } 800 \text{ g} = 40 \text{ g}$$

Step 2. *Determine the total number of Calories from the protein hydrolysate.*

$$40 \text{ g} \times 4 \text{ Cal/g} = 160 \text{ Cal}$$

Step 3. *Determine the number of grams of glucose.*

$$50\% \text{ of } 150 \text{ g} = 75 \text{ g}$$

Step 4. *Determine the number of Calories from the glucose.*

$$75 \text{ g} \times 4 \text{ Cal/g} = 300 \text{ Cal}$$

Step 5. *Add the number of Calories from the protein hydrolysate to the number of Calories from the glucose.*

$$160 \text{ Cal} + 300 \text{ Cal} = 460 \text{ Cal}$$

In each of the following problems determine (a) the number of Calories being administered, and (b) the rate at which the IV should be administered.

1.

IV ORDER
Name: ROBINSON EMILIE   **RM–BD:** 337–2
1,000 ML 10% GLUCOSE   6 HR

(The drop factor is 15.)

2.

IV ORDER
Name: BERGSTROM, ERIC   **RM–BD:** 200–A AGE 3
120 ML 5% GLUCOSE   4 HR

(The drop factor is 60.)

3.

IV ORDER
Name: BILKER, BRIAN   **RM–BD:** 559–3
750 ML 10% FRUCTOSE   4 HR

(The drop factor is 15.)

4.

IV ORDER
Name: TRUETT, MADELINE   **RM–BD:** 436–C AGE 2
80 ML 6% DEXTRAN   4 HR

(The drop factor is 60.)

5. A patient was given 500 ml of solution IV in 8 hours. The solution contained 300 ml of 5% protein hydrolysate, 150 ml of 40% glucose, and 50 ml of saline solution. How many Calories were administered? What should be the rate of flow? The drop factor is 15.

6. A patient is given 1,000 ml of 10% fructose solution in sodium chloride solution IV in 6 hours. How many Calories were administered? What should be the rate of administration? The drop factor is 15.

7. An infant is given 100 ml IV in 4 hours. The solution contains 70 ml of 5% protein hydrolysate, 10 ml of 50% glucose, and 20 ml of saline solution. How many Calories were administered and what was the rate of administration? The drop factor is 60.

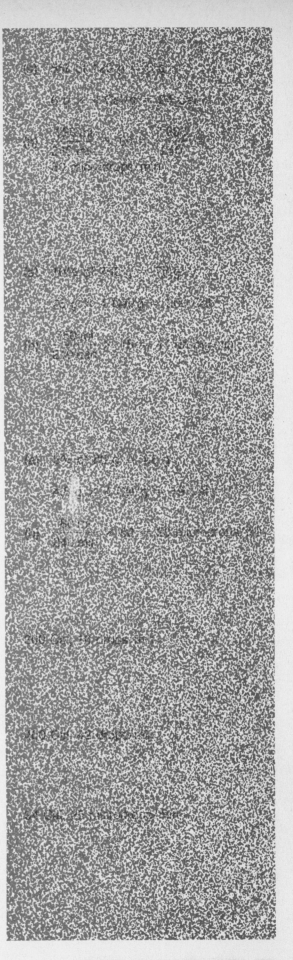

8. A patient is given 500 ml 6% dextran solution IV in 4 hours. How many Calories were administered and at what rate? The drop factor is 15.

9. A patient was given 1,000 ml IV in 5 hours. The solution contained 600 ml 6% protein hydrolysate and 400 ml saline solution. How many Calories were administered? What was the rate of administration? The drop factor is 15.

10. A patient was given 1,000 ml IV in 8 hours. The solution contained 400 ml 5% protein hydrolysate, 200 ml 50% glucose, 100 ml 10% fructose, and 300 ml saline solution. How many Calories were administered? What was the rate of administration? The drop factor is 15.

Passing score is no more than *1* error.

Chapter 18

Milliequivalents (mEq's)

Section 1   Intravenous Medications Involving Milliequivalents

Frequently, medications in milliequivalent amounts are added directly to IV fluids. mEq (or MEQ) is the abbreviation for milliequivalent.

Consider the following order:

IV ORDER		
Name: WATSON, JUNE		**RM–BD:** 108–2
Solution	**Time**	**Available Medication**
1,000 ML NORMAL SALINE + 40 MEQ KCL	8 HR	2 MEQ/1.0 ML

The nurse, or pharmacist, must calculate the amount of medication to use according to the following equation:

$$\frac{\text{Desired amount}}{\text{Available amount}} = \frac{\text{How much we are going to use}}{\text{How much we have on hand}}$$

Answer the following questions.

1. What is the desired amount of potassium chloride?

2. What is the available amount of potassium chloride?

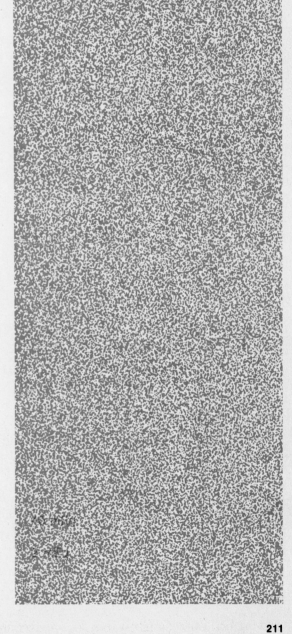

3. At this time, do you know how much we are going to use?

4. How much do we have on hand?

5. Using the equation, calculate how much solution we are going to use.

6. Assume that ampuls of potassium chloride are available in 10-ml, 20-ml, or 30-ml sizes.

What size ampul should be selected?

7. The order indicates that the KCl is to be administered IV. What must be done with the 20 ml of KCl solution before it is administered to the patient?

Consider the following order:

IV ORDER		
Name: TOPPER, CHARLES		**RM–BD:** 216–A
Solution	**Time**	**Available Medication**
1,000 ML 5% D/W + 48 MEQ KCL	6 HR	3.2 MEQ/1.0 ML

8. Use the following equation to determine the amount of potassium chloride to be added to the IV fluid.

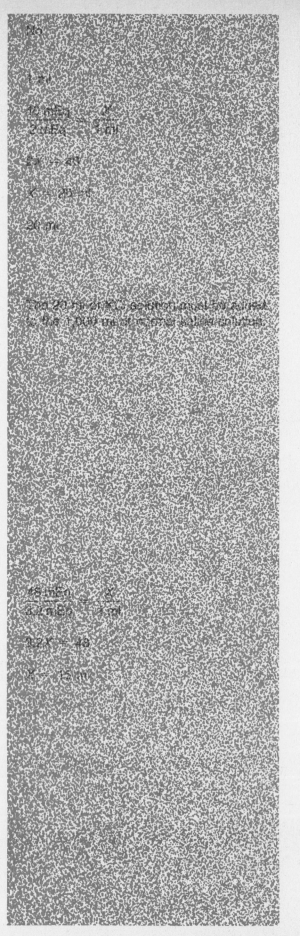

$$\frac{\text{Desired amount}}{\text{Available amount}} = \frac{\text{How much are we going to use}}{\text{How much we have on hand}}$$

For each of the following orders, calculate the amount of medication to be injected into the IV bottle.

9.

IV ORDER		
Name: KELSON, MARY		**RM–BD:** 317–C
Solution	**Time**	**Available Medication**
1,000 ML 5% D/W + 22.3 MEQ SO- DIUM BICARBONATE	8 HR	44.6 MEQ/50 ML

10.

IV ORDER		
Name: PURCELL, JAMES		**RM–BD:** 602–1
Solution	**Time**	**Available Medication**
1,000 ML N/S + 17 MEQ MAGNESIUM SULFATE	6 HR	81.2 MEQ/100 ML

11.

IV ORDER		
Name: QUANDE, ENID		**RM–BD:** 1012
Solution	**Time**	**Available Medication**
1,000 ML 5% D/W + 44.6 MEQ SODIUM BICARBONATE	8 HR	44.6 MEQ/50 ML

12.

IV ORDER		
Name: STOVELL, HENRY		**RM–BD:** 330–D
Solution	**Time**	**Available Medication**
1,000 ML N/S + 2 MEQ CALCIUM CHLORIDE	8 HR	1.36 MEQ/1.0 ML

13.

IV ORDER		
Name: SUZANNE, RUTH		**RM–BD:** 138–1
Solution	**Time**	**Available Medication**
1,000 ML 5% D/W + 8.5 MEQ MAGNESIUM SULFATE	6 HR	81.2 MEQ/100 ML

14.

IV ORDER		
Name: WILSON, MARGUERITE		**RM–BD:** 404–B
Solution	**Time**	**Available Medication**
1,000 ML N/S + 18 MEQ CALCIUM GLUCEPTATE	8 HR	0.9 MEQ/1.0 ML

15.

IV ORDER		
Name: DOBSON, FRED		**RM–BD:** 111–1
Solution	**Time**	**Available Medication**
1,000 ML 5% D/W + 9 MEQ CALCIUM GLUCONATE	8 HR	0.45 MEQ/1.0 ML

Passing score is no more than *2* errors.

Section 2   Oral Medications Involving Milliequivalents

When a medication in milliequivalents is given orally, it is usually administered in divided dosages. The nurse may have to calculate the amount of medication to be given per dose. Consider the following order:

60 mEq potassium chloride per 24 hours, to be given in 3 doses.

Dividing the total dosage (60 mEq) by the number of doses (3) = 20 mEq per dose. The following formula is used to determine the amount of medication to be given per dose.

$$\frac{\text{Desired amount}}{\text{Available amount}} = \frac{\text{How much we are going to use}}{\text{How much we have on hand}}$$

Assume that the following is available:

Potassium chloride, 20 mEq/15 ml

Try to answer the following questions:

1. Assume you are trying to determine the amount of medication to give per dose. What is the desired amount?

2. What is the available amount?

3. Do you know the amount to use?

4. What is the amount on hand?

5. Use the formula to determine the amount per dose.

6. How should this medication be administered?

   Consider the following:

   Order: 80 mEq potassium chloride per day in 4 doses.
   Available: potassium chloride, 40 mEq/30 ml

7. What is the mEq value per dose?

8. Determine the amount of medication to be given per dose.

Consider the following order:

Name: PERKINS, HELENE	**RM–BD:** 369–B
Medication Order	**Available Medication**
20 MEQ CALCIUM CHLORIDE QID	40 MEQ/30 ML

9. What is the desired amount?

10. What is the available amount?

11. What is the amount we are going to use?

12. What is the amount we have on hand?

13. Determine the amount we are going to use.

14. How often should this medication be administered?

15. How should this medication be administered?

16. If this medication is administered at home, how much would you tell the patient to take for each dose?

Passing score is no more than *1* error.

Section 3   Changing Per Cent Solutions to mEq/ml

If a medication is available as a per cent solution, calculate the number of milliequivalents per milliliter.

Example: *Calcium chloride is available as a 10% solution. Calculate the number of milliequivalents per milliliter.*

In order to determine the milliequivalent, you need to know the molecular weight of the compound as well as the ionic charges. Both are usually stated on the label. For example:

The molecular weight of calcium chloride = 147

When an element has an ionic charge, the charge will also be indicated on the label. Let's consider an example.

As you may know from your chemistry courses, Ca is the symbol for calcium.

Ca^{2+} means that calcium has an ionic charge of 2.

Let's consider another example.

The symbol for magnesium is Mg. Mg^{2+} means that magnesium has an ionic charge of 2.

When the charge is 1, the symbol will simply show a plus sign. For example, K is the symbol for potassium. *K^+ means that potassium has an ionic charge of 1.*

Sometimes, the charge may be shown as a minus sign. For example, Cl is the symbol for chloride. *Cl^- means that chloride has an ionic charge of −1.*

For the purpose of determining the milliequivalent of a solution, both a plus sign and a minus sign mean that the ionic charge is 1.

In each of the following examples, determine the ionic charge.

1. Chloride Cl^-

2. Magnesium Mg^{2+}

3. Bicarbonate HCO_3^-

4. Calcium Ca^{2+}

When a medication is available in a per cent solution, the following formula is used to determine the number of milliequivalents per milliliter.

$$\frac{\% \text{ of the solution} \times 10 \times \text{ionic charge}}{\text{Molecular weight}} = \frac{\text{Number of}}{\text{mEq/ml}}$$

Consider the following example:

Potassium chloride, KCl, is available as a 15% solution. The molecular weight of KCl is 74.6. Try to answer the following questions.

5. What is the per cent of the solution?

6. If the symbol for the potassium ion is K^+, what is the ionic charge?

7. What is the molecular weight of potassium chloride?

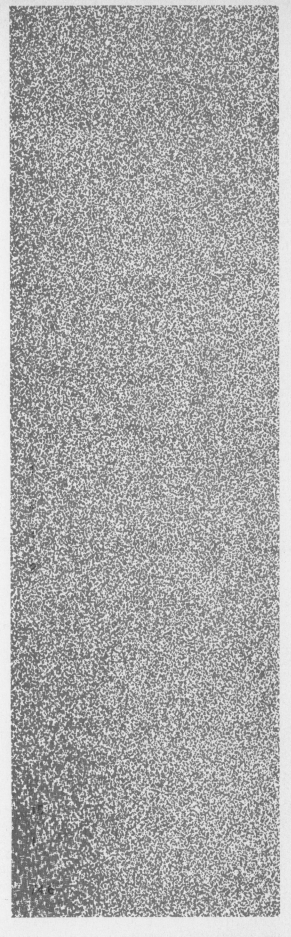

8. Using the above equation, determine the number of milli-equivalents per milliliter.

In each of the following examples, determine the number of mEq/ml. Express the result to 2 decimal places.

9. Calcium gluconate, molecular weight 448, is available as a 10% solution. How many mEq Ca^{2+} are present per ml?

10. Calcium chloride is available as a 10% solution. The molecular weight is 147. How many mEq Ca^{2+}/ml?

11. Potassium chloride, molecular weight 74.6, is available as a 24% solution. How many mEq K^+/ml?

12. Magnesium sulfate, molecular weight 246, is available as a 10% solution. How many mEq Mg^{2+}/ml?

13. Calcium gluceptate, molecular weight 490, is available as a 23% solution. How many mEq Ca^{2+}/ml?

14. Calcium levulinate, molecular weight 288, is available as a 10% solution. How many mEq Ca^{2+}/ml?

Passing score is no more than *1* error.

Section 4   Changing Milligrams to Milliequivalents

If a medication is available in tablet form, you may have to change milligrams of drug to milliequivalents of the same drug. Consider the following example.

Potassium phenoxymethyl penicillin, molecular weight 388, is available in 250-mg tablets. How many milliequivalents K^+ per tablet?

The following formula is used:

$$\frac{\text{No. of milligrams} \times \text{ionic charge}}{\text{Molecular weight}} = \text{No. of mEq}$$

1. Using the above formula, calculate the number of mEq K^+ per table.

In the above formula, the amount of drug must be expressed in milligrams. Therefore, if the order is expressed in grams, you must first convert grams to milligrams. Consider the following example.

Order: Give 6 g potassium chloride per day. Molecular weight 74.6. Determine the number of milliequivalents of K^+ in the 6-g dose.

Answer the following questions:

2. In order to use the above equation, how must the amount of drug be expressed?

3. How many milligrams is 6 g?

4. Using the formula, determine the number of mEq K^+ in a 6-g dose.

5. If this medication is to be given q.i.d., how many grams of medication should be given per dose?

6. If this medication is to be given q.i.d., how many milliequivalents should be given per dose?

In each of the following examples, calculate the number of milliequivalents in the given amount of drug.

7. Calcium lactate is available in 600-mg tablets. Molecular weight = 308. How many mEq Ca^{2+} per tablet?

8. 1,000-mg calcium carbonate tablets, molecular weight 100, contain how many mEq Ca^{2+}?

9. 500-mg calcium gluconate tablets, molecular weight 448, contain how many mEq Ca^{2+}?

Passing score is no more than *1* error.

Unit Two—Practice Tests

The following end-of-unit tests are designed to test your mastery of the subject matter in Chapters 10–18. There are four tests. Answers are provided for Tests 1 and 2, and the student should follow the usual Reinforced Learning procedures. Tests 3 and 4 are without answers and may be used in the classroom.

Unit Two   Practice Test No. 1

1. a) 210 pounds = _____ kg
   b) 6′4″ = _____ cm
   c) 98.2°F = _____°C
   d) 1 teaspoonful = _____ ml
   e) 10 drops = _____ ml

2. a) 300 mcg = _____ mg
   b) 0.2 mg = _____ mcg
   c) 1.5 mg = _____ g
   d) 67.9 kg = _____ lb
   e) 0.5 liter = _____ ml

3. a) 25 cm = _____ m
   b) 1.5 g = _____ mg
   c) 125 cm = _____ in.
   d) 375 mcg = _____ mg
   e) 2 ml = _____ cc

4. A patient's weight, height, and temperature were recorded as 198 lb, 5′, and 104°F respectively. What were these figures in kg, cm, and °C?

For questions 5–9 calculate the number of tablets or capsules to be administered.

5.

Name: WALTERS, LORI	RM–BD: 367−2
Medication Order	**Available Medication**
ASCORBIC ACID 1,000 MG	TABLETS 0.5 G

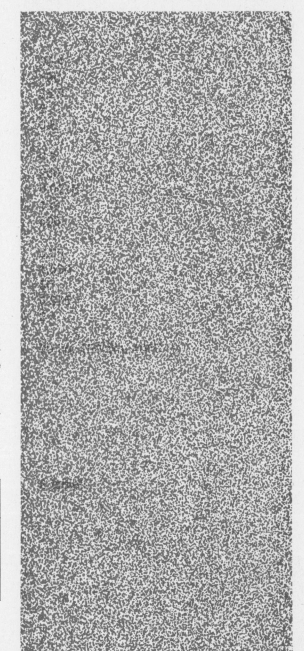

6.

Name: MIRELLES, JUAN	RM–BD: 209-1
Medication Order	**Available Medication**
SYNTHROID 0.2 MG	TABLETS 200 MCG

7.

Name: MAXWELL, FRED	RM–BD: 1427-C
Medication Order	**Available Medication**
TERRAMYCIN 250 MG	CAPSULES 125 MG

8.

Name: BROADWELL, LEWIS	RM–BD: 502-A
Medication Order	**Available Medication**
DIGOXIN 250 MCG	TABLETS 0.25 MG

9.

Name: HENDRICKS, FLORA	RM–BD: 446-4
Medication Order	**Available Medication**
GANTRISIN 1 G QID	TABLETS 500 MG

Write statements for the following orders.

10.

Name: ZOBEL, ANDREW	RM–BD: 763-2
Medication Order	**Available Medication**
THIAMINE 75 MG IM QD	0.1 G/1.0 ML

11. How would you give 25 U of insulin from a U 100 bottle using a tuberculin syringe?

12.

Name: ALBERTSON, PAUL	**RM–BD:** 305–C

Medication Order	**Available Medication**
POTASSIUM CHLORIDE 20 MEQ QID	40 MEQ/30 ML

13.

Name: MONROE, CLAUDE	**RM–BD:** 621–1

Medication Order	**Available Medication**
SODIUM AMPICILLIN 0.8 G IM Q6H	1 G

Directions for reconstitution

ADD 2.4 ML STERILE WATER.
RECONSTITUTED SOLUTION WILL CONTAIN
400 MG/1.0 ML AND MUST BE USED WITHIN
1 HOUR.

14.

Name: NORDHOFF, PHYLLIS	**RM–BD:** 625–1
Wt. in kg. 41.7	

Medication Order	**Available Medication**
TETRACYCLINE HYDROCHLORIDE Q6H	125 MG/5 ML

Pediatric Dosage

12 MG/KG/DAY

15.

Name: DIXON, ALEX	RM–BD: 402–1
Medication Order	**Available Medication**
PENICILLIN G 500,000 U IM Q4H	5,000,000 U
Directions for reconstitution ADD 18 ML STERILE WATER TO PROVIDE A CONCENTRATION OF 250,000 U/1 ML.	

16.

Name: PARSONS, WAYNE	RM–BD: 893–1
Medication Order	**Available Medication**
MORPHINE SULFATE 8 MG SUBQ PRN	10 MG/1.0 ML

17.

Name: BRUBAKER, PHYLLIS	RM–BD: 1011–3
Wt. in kg. 7.5	
Medication Order	**Available Medication**
KANAMYCIN SULFATE IM BID	75 MG/2 ML
Pediatric Dosage 15 MG/KG/DAY	

18.

Name: CLEVELAND, ELENA	RM–BD: 104–1

Medication Order	Available Medication
STREPTOMYCIN 0.5 G IM BID	5 G

Directions for reconstitution

ADD 6.5 ML STERILE WATER.
RECONSTITUTED SOLUTION WILL CONTAIN
500 MG/1 ML. STORE IN REFRIGERATOR FOR
NOT MORE THAN 14 DAYS.

19.

Name: RUDOLPH, JO–ANN	RM–BD: 603–1

Medication Order	Available Medication
KCL 20 MEQ QAM	40 MEQ/30 ML

If the patient is to take this medication at home, how much should be taken?

20.

Name: ROSENBERG, PAUL	RM–BD: 206–3
Wt. in kg. 16.0	

Medication Order	Available Medication
ERYTHROMYCIN SULFATE QID	400 MG/5 ML

Pediatric Dosage

50 MG/KG/DAY

21.

Name: PORTERFIELD, LINNEA	RM–BD: 382–A

Medication Order	**Available Medication**
TICARCILLIN DISODIUM 0.8 G IM BID	3 G

Directions for reconstitution

ADD 6 ML STERILE WATER. RECONSTITUTED SOLUTION WILL CONTAIN 1 G/2.5 ML AND IS STABLE FOR 24 HOURS AT ROOM TEMPERATURE OR FOR 72 HOURS IF REFRIGERATED.

22.

Name: WOJCIK, THAD	RM–BD: 337–2

Medication Order	**Available Medication**
MAGNESIUM SULFATE 5G HS	20%

23.

Name: VALENTINE, JUDY	RM–BD: 650–4
Wt. in kg. 6.0	

Medication Order	**Available Medication**
GARAMYCIN IM Q8H	10 MG/1.0 ML

Pediatric Dosage

7.5 MG/KG/DAY

24.

Name: STONE, MARLENE	RM–BD: 603–A

Medication Order	Available Medication
PENICILLIN 500,000 U IM QID	5,000,000 U

Directions for reconstitution

ADD 23 ML, 18 ML, 8 ML, OR 3 ML
STERILE WATER TO PROVIDE A
CONCENTRATION OF 200,000 U, 250,000 U,
500,000 U, OR 1,000,000 U/1 ML
RESPECTIVELY.

- a) Which of the above concentrations should you select?
- b) How much sterile water should you add to the vial?
- c) How much reconstituted solution should you give the patient?
- d) How should you relabel the vial?

25.

Name: DUPONT, CHARLENE	RM–BD: 504–3

Medication Order	Available Medication
VITAMIN B$_{12}$ 400 MCG IM QD	1,000 MCG/1.0 ML

26.

Name: TURNER, LISA	RM–BD: 460–A

Medication Order	Available Medication
PENICILLIN G 250,000 U IM Q4H	1,000,000 U

Directions for reconstitution

ADD 9.6 ML STERILE WATER.
RECONSTITUTED SOLUTION WILL CONTAIN
100,000 U/ML AND IS STABLE FOR 1 WEEK
UNDER REFRIGERATION

27.

Name: PARKER, EUGENE	RM–BD: 118–3
Medication Order	**Available Medication**
KCL 40 MEQ QD	40 MEQ/15 ML

28.

Name: PRESTON, HENRI	RM–BD: 1653–4
Medication Order	**Available Medication**
LANOXIN 250 MCG IM Q6H	0.5 MG/2 CC

29.

Name: BRISCOE, EMILY	RM–BD: 903–1
Medication Order	**Available Medication**
EPINEPHRINE 0.5 MG SUBQ STAT	1:1,000

30.

Name: BRIXTON, TIMOTHY	RM–BD: 302–3
Medication Order	**Available Medication**
200,000 U PENICILLIN G IM QID	5,000,000 U

Directions for reconstitution

ADD 23 ML, 18 ML, 8 ML, OR 3 ML STERILE WATER TO PROVIDE 200,000 U, 250,000 U, 500,000 U, OR 1,000,000 U/1.0 ML RESPECTIVELY.

31.

Name: ROBINSON, JANINE	RM–BD: 305–2
Medication Order	**Available Medication**
MEPERIDINE HYDROCHLORIDE 100 MG IM PRN	0.05 G/1 ML

Calculate the rate of flow of the following IV orders.

32.

IV ORDER	
Name: CUSTER, JOAN	RM–BD: 336–2
1,200 ML 5% GLUCOSE 6 HR	

(The drop factor is 10.)

33.

IV ORDER	
Name: BENSON, IRVING	RM–BD: 540–A
100 ML 10% GLUCOSE 3 HR	

(The drop factor is 60 microdrops/ml.)

34.

IV ORDER	
Name: SUTROW, AGNES	RM–BD: 390–C
900 ML 5% D/W 6 HR	

(The drop factor is 12.)

35.

IV ORDER	
Name: SENECA, IRIS	**RM–BD:** 404–4
1,200 ML PHYSIOLOGIC SALINE 6 HR	

(The drop factor is 15.)

36.

IV ORDER	
Name: KLAUS, PAMELA	**RM–BD:** 721–1
300 ML 10% GLUCOSE 8 HR	

(The drop factor is 60 microdrops/ml.)

For the following problems calculate the original rate of IV flow, and also the revised rate of flow at the beginning of the next shift.

37.

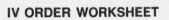

IV ORDER WORKSHEET

NAME: Blakestone, Arnold	RM–BD: 305–4				
			AMT LEFT AT END OF SHIFT		
	TIME START	TIME END	0700	1500	2300
1,000 ml 10% glucose 8 hr	1800	0200		400	

(The drop factor is 15.)

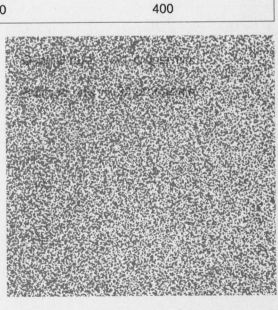

38.

IV ORDER WORKSHEET

NAME: Simmons, Gwen		RM–BD: 431–1			
	TIME START	TIME END	AMT LEFT AT END OF SHIFT		
			0700	1500	2300
1,200 ml 5% D/W 8 hr	0800	1600	175		

(The drop factor is 10.)

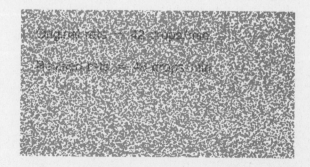

39.

IV ORDER WORKSHEET

NAME: Browning, Alma		RM–BD: 407–1			
	TIME START	TIME END	AMT LEFT AT END OF SHIFT		
			0700	1500	2300
900 ml physiologic saline 6 hr	1200	1800	500		

(The drop factor is 12.)

40.

IV ORDER WORKSHEET

NAME: Holmes, Richard		RM–BD: 101–4			
	TIME START	TIME END	AMT LEFT AT END OF SHIFT		
			0700	1500	2300
2,000 ml 5% D/W 12 hr	0900	2100	1100		

(The drop factor is 15.)

41.

IV ORDER WORKSHEET

NAME: Princeton, Melvin	RM–BD: 229–4				

	TIME START	TIME END	AMT LEFT AT END OF SHIFT		
			0700	1500	2300
500 ml 5% D/W 4 hr	2200	0200		400	

(The drop factor is 12.)

For the following orders calculate the amount of medication to be added to the IV bottle and also the rate of IV flow, assuming that the volume of IV fluid is not changed by the addition of the medication.

42.

IV ORDER

Name: SANDERSON, EDMUND   **RM–BD:** 521–3

Solution	Time	Available Medication
1,000 ML N/S + 27 MEQ CALCIUM GLUCONATE	8 HR	0.45 MEQ/1.0 ML

(The drop factor is 12.)

43.

IV ORDER

Name: MOREHEAD, SYBIL   **RM–BD:** 346–1

Solution	Time	Available Medication
1,000 ML 5% D/W + 30 MEQ KCL	8 HR	2 MEQ/1.0 ML

(The drop factor is 15.)

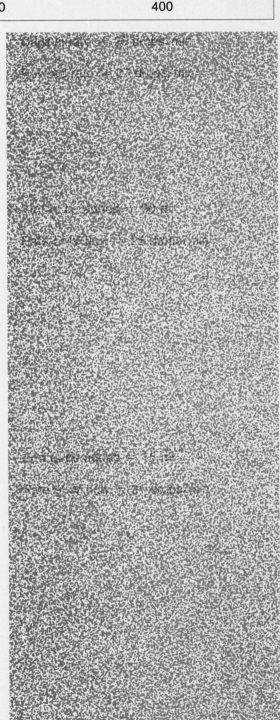

44.

IV ORDER		
Name: TYLER, VICKI		**RM–BD:** 1612–D
Solution	**Time**	**Available Medication**
500 ML N/S + 18 MEQ CALCIUM GLUCONATE	8 HR	0.9 MEQ/1.0 ML

(The drop factor is 10.)

45.

IV ORDER		
Name: WASHINGTON, WANDA		**RM–BD:** 204–A
Solution	**Time**	**Available Medication**
1,000 ML N/S + 22.3 MEQ SODIUM BICARBONATE	8 HR	44.6 MEQ/50 ML

(The drop factor is 15.)

46.

IV ORDER		
Name: LINCOLN, MARLA		**RM–BD:** 118–C
Solution	**Time**	**Available Medication**
1,000 ML N/S + 2 MEQ CALCIUM CHLORIDE	12 HR	1.36 MEQ/1.0 ML

(The drop factor is 12.)

For the following orders, calculate the rate of flow of the piggybacks, and also the rate of IV flow between piggybacks.

47.

IV ORDER	
Name: PARKER, ARTHUR	**RM–BD:** 700–2
2,000 ML 5% D/W 24 HR	

Name: PARKER, ARTHUR		**RM–BD:** 700–2
Medication Order	**Time**	**Available Medication**
AMPICILLIN 1 G IVPB Q6H	30 MIN	1.0 G
Directions		
DISSOLVE IN 50 ML 5% D/W		

(The drop factor is 15.)

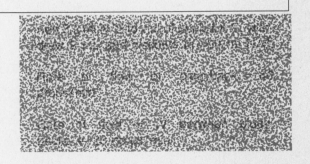

48.

IV ORDER	
Name: PETERS, TRACEY	**RM–BD:** 870–4
2,000 ML N/S 16 HR	

Name: PETERS, TRACEY		**RM–BD:** 870–4
Medication Order	**Time**	**Available Medication**
PENICILLIN G 1,000,000 U IVPB Q4H	30 MIN	5,000,000 U
Directions for Reconstitution		
Add 8.2 ML DILUENT TO PROVIDE A CONCENTRATION OF 500,000 U/1.0 ML.		
Directions for Piggyback		
DISSOLVE IN 100 ML N/S.		

(The drop factor is 12.)

49.

IV ORDER	
Name: MILLER, DALIA	**RM–BD:** 403–1
2,000 ML 5% D/W 24 HR	

Name: MILLER, DALIA		**RM–BD:** 403–1
Medication Order	**Time**	**Available Medication**
KEFLIN 500 MG IVPB Q4H	1 HR	500 MG/100 ML 5% D/W

(The drop factor is 10.)

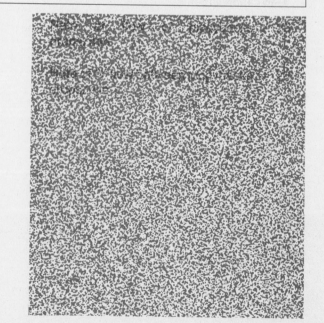

50.

IV ORDER	
Name: SPIEGEL, BEN	**RM–BD:** 206–A
2,500 ML N/S 24 HR	

Name: SPIEGEL, BEN		**RM–BD:** 206–A
Medication Order	**Time**	**Available Medication**
CHLORAMPHENICOL 500 MG IVPB Q6H	30 MIN	500 MG/50 ML N/S

(The drop factor is 15.)

51.

IV ORDER	
Name: CROWN, SPENCER	**RM–BD:** 431–C
1,200 ML PHYSIOLOGIC SALINE 18 HR	

Name: CROWN, SPENCER		**RM–BD:** 431–C
Medication Order	**Time**	**Available Medication**
GENTAMICIN 120 MG IVPB Q6H	30 MIN	80 MG/2 ML
Directions		
DISSOLVE IN 100 ML PHYSIOLOGIC SALINE.		

(The drop factor is 15.)

How long will the IV flow in the following orders?

52.

IV ORDER	
Name: FROMER, BETTY	**RM–BD:** 627–2
1,500 ML 5% D/W 50 DROPS/MIN	

(The drop factor is 15.)

53.

IV ORDER	
Name: ALLWYN, LOUISA	**RM–BD:** 322–D
900 ML PHYSIOLOGIC SALINE 35 DROPS/MIN	

(The drop factor is 12.)

54.

IV ORDER	
Name: TWILEY, JAMES	**RM–BD:** 552–2
800 ML 5% GLUCOSE 40 DROPS/MIN	

(The drop factor is 15.)

55.

IV ORDER	
Name: HALL, BART	**RM–BD:** 740–1
200 ML 10% GLUCOSE 50 MICRODROPS/MIN	

(The drop factor is 60.)

56.

IV ORDER	
Name: GROSSEL, CHESTER	**RM–BD:** 126–3
1,000 ML 5% D/W 25 DROPS/MIN	

(The drop factor is 12.)

57.

IV ORDER	
Name: RIVERWOOD, ALBERT	**RM–BD:** 205–3
1,200 ML 5% D/W 150 ML/HR	

58.

IV ORDER	
Name: KOWALSKI, PIERRE	**RM–BD:** 312–4
800 ML PHYSIOLOGIC SALINE 100 ML/HR	

59.

IV ORDER
Name: KRAFT, IRENE   **RM–BD:** 403–4
100 ML 5% GLUCOSE   25 ML/HR

60. What will be the rate of IV flow in question #57 if the drop factor is 15?

61. What will be the rate of IV flow in question #58 if the drop factor is 12?

62. What will be the rate of IV flow in question #59 if the drop factor is 60?

63. 0.85% sodium chloride solution contains how many mEq Na^+ per ml? Molecular weight = 58.5.

64. An infant was given 120 ml of 6% dextran (a carbohydrate) IV in 6 hours. How many Calories did the infant receive?

65. How many milliequivalents of Ca^{2+} per milliliter are in a 5% solution of calcium chloride, molecular weight 147?

66. An infant was given 120 ml IV in 4 hours. The solution contained 80 ml of 5% protein hydrolysate, 20 ml of 50% glucose solution, and 20 ml saline. How many Calories were administered?

67. Magnesium sulfate, molecular weight 246, is available as a 50% solution. How many mEq Mg^{2+} per ml?

68. A patient was given 1,000 ml of solution IV in 8 hours. The solution contained 600 ml of 5% protein hydrolysate, 300 ml of 50% glucose solution, and 100 ml of saline solution. How many Calories were administered?

69. How many mEq Ca^{2+} are present in a 500-mg calcium carbonate tablet? Molecular weight of calcium carbonate is 100.

70. A patient was given 1,000 ml IV in 12 hours. The IV fluid contained 500 ml of 10% dextrose, 300 ml of 5% protein hydrolysate, and 200 ml of normal saline. How many Calories were administered?

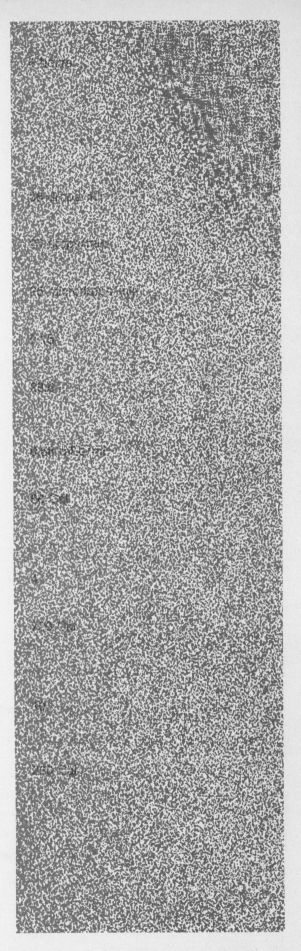

Unit Two   Practice Test No. 2

1. a) 120 cm = _____ m
   b) 0.02 g = _____ mg
   c) 0.05 liters = _____ ml
   d) 0.03 mg = _____ mcg
   e) 40 in. = _____ cm

2. a) 120 pounds = _____ kg
   b) 4′10″ = _____ cm
   c) 97.8°F = _____ °C
   d) 1 tablespoonful = _____ ml
   e) 0.25 ml = _____ drops

3. a) 0.1 g = _____ mg
   b) 100 mcg = _____ mg
   c) 0.1% of 500 g = _____ g
   d) 40.6 cc = _____ ml
   e) 2 teaspoonfuls = _____ ml

4. A patient's weight, temperature, and height were recorded as 140 pounds, 100.8° F, and 5′4″. Convert these figures to a) kg, b) °C, and c) cm.

For questions 5–9 calculate the number of tablets to be administered.

5.

Name: BLOCHER, TRICIA	RM–BD: 124–2
Medication Order	**Available Medication**
DEXAMETHASONE 750 MCG	TABLETS 0.25 MG

6.

Name: ROCHESTER, CHRISTINA	RM–BD: 213–1
Medication Order	**Available Medication**
ASPIRIN 0.65 G	TABLETS 325 MG

7.

Name: MAXIME, HAROLD	RM–BD: 326–A
Medication Order	**Available Medication**
SYNTHROID 0.1 MG	TABLETS 100 MCG

8.

Name: CLIFTON, WARREN	RM–BD: 321–3
Medication Order	**Available Medication**
HALDOL 250 MCG	TABLETS 0.5 MG

9.

Name: TRAXLER, LUCILLE	RM–BD: 641–D
Medication Order	**Available Medication**
WARFARIN SODIUM 10 MG	TABLETS 5 MG

Write statements for the following orders.

10.

Name: LECLAIRE, HENRY	RM–BD: 308–B
Medication Order	**Available Medication**
THIAMINE 0.03 G IM QD	100 MG/1.0 ML

11.

Name: BRIXTON, CHERYL	RM–BD: 762–1
Wt. in kg. 33.3	
Medication Order	**Available Medication**
TETRACYCLINE QID	125 MG/5 ML
Pediatric Dosage	
30 MG/KG/DAY	

12.

Name: COMPTON, SOPHIA	RM–BD: 204-2

Medication Order	Available Medication
PENICILLIN G 500,000 U IM Q4H	5,000,000 U

Directions for reconstitution

ADD 18 ML STERILE WATER. RECONSTITUTED SOLUTION WILL CONTAIN 250,000 U/1.0 ML AND IS STABLE FOR 1 WEEK UNDER REFRIGERATION.

13.

Name: MARSHALL, LORI	RM–BD: 193-C
Wt. in kg. 25.0	

Medication Order	Available Medication
TETRACYCLINE HYDROCHLORIDE Q8H	125 MG/5 ML

Pediatric Dosage

15 MG/KG/DAY

14.

Name: CZOKER, ELLEN	RM–BD: 451-C

Medication Order	Available Medication
VITAMIN B_{12} 15 MCG IM QD	30 MCG/1.0 ML

15.

Name: BARLOW, SYLVIA	RM–BD: 112–D

Medication Order	Available Medication
PENICILLIN 400,000 U IM Q4H	2,000,000 U

Directions for reconstitution

ADD 9 ML STERILE WATER. RECONSTITUTED SOLUTION WILL CONTAIN 200,000 U/1.0 ML. STORE IN REFRIGERATOR.

16.

Name: HARPER, DAVID	RM–BD: 432–1

Medication Order	Available Medication
KCL 10 MEQ QAM	40 MEQ/30 ML

17.

Name: BAILEY, ANDREW	RM–BD: 209–3
Wt. in kg. 8.0	

Medication Order	Available Medication
KANAMYCIN IM BID	75 MG/2 ML

Pediatric Dosage

15 MG/KG/DAY

18.

Name: CONNI, SERENA	RM–BD: 219–3

Medication Order	Available Medication
HYDROXYZINE HYDROCHLORIDE 100 MG IM PRN	50 MG/1.0 ML

19.

Name: WEST, HOMER	RM–BD: 341–1

Medication Order	Available Medication
STREPTOMYCIN 200 MG IM Q6H	1.0 G

Directions for reconstitution

ADD 4.5 ML STERILE WATER. RECONSTITUTED SOLUTION WILL CONTAIN 200 MG/1.0 ML. STORE IN REFRIGERATOR FOR NO MORE THAN 14 DAYS.

20.

Name: GOMBERG, ALBERT	RM–BD: 202–4

Medication Order	Available Medication
INSULIN 60 U SUBQ (USE A TUBERCULIN SYRINGE)	100 U/1.0 ML

21.

Name: FLACK, LESTER	RM–BD: 540–A
Wt. in kg. 15.0	

Medication Order	Available Medication
ISONIAZID IM QAM	100 MG/1.0 ML

Pediatric Dosage

10 MG/KG/DAY

22.

Name: HUGHES, CINDY	RM–BD: 201–C
Medication Order	**Available Medication**
SODIUM AMPICILLIN 750 MG IM Q6H	1 G
Directions for reconstitution	
ADD 2.4 ML STERILE WATER. RECONSTITUTED LIQUID WILL CONTAIN 400 MG/1.0 ML AND MUST BE USED WITHIN 1 HOUR.	

23.

Name: CRAWFORD, MARK	RM–BD: 337–2
Medication Order	**Available Medication**
EPINEPHRINE 1 MG SUBQ STAT	1:1,000

24.

Name: ROCKFORD, SHELLEY	RM–BD: 334–1
Medication Order	**Available Medication**
KCL 40 MEQ BID	20 MEQ/15 ML

25.

Name: KASS, GUSTAVE	RM–BD: 873–C
Medication Order	**Available Medication**
MAGNESIUM SULFATE 10 G HS	20%

26.

Name: WABASH, FRITZ	RM–BD: 154–2
Medication Order	**Available Medication**
MORPHINE SULFATE 7.5 MG SUBQ PRN	15 MG/1.0 ML

27.

Name: STREATOR, BRENDA	RM–BD: 118–C

Medication Order	Available Medication
AMPICILLIN TRIHYDRATE 500 MG QID	5.0 G

Directions for reconstitution

ADD 70 ML WATER. RECONSTITUTED SOLUTION WILL CONTAIN 250 MG/5 ML AND IS STABLE FOR 14 DAYS WHEN REFRIGERATED.

28.

Name: BISMARK, HELENE	RM–BD: 240–1

Medication Order	Available Medication
LANOXIN 200 MCG IM Q6H	0.5 MG/2 CC

29.

Name: BARNEY, MARTIN	RM–BD: 430–2

Medication Order	Available Medication
PENICILLIN 500,000 U IM Q4H	5,000,000 U

Directions for reconstitution

ADD 18 ML STERILE WATER. RECONSTITUTED SOLUTION WILL CONTAIN 250,000 U/1.0 ML AND IS STABLE FOR 1 WEEK WHEN REFRIGERATED.

30.

Name: PERKINS, HERBERT	RM–BD: 304–D

Medication Order	Available Medication
MEPERIDINE HYDROCHLORIDE 75 MG IM PRN	0.05 G/1.0 ML

31.

Name: EVERSON, DALE	**RM–BD:** 300–1

Medication Order	**Available Medication**
PENICILLIN G 250,000 U IM QID	5,000,000 U

Directions for reconstitution

ADD 23 ML, 18 ML, 8 ML, OR 3 ML
STERILE WATER TO PROVIDE A
CONCENTRATION OF 200,000 U/1.0 ML,
250,000 U/1.0 ML, 500,000 U/1.0 ML, OR
1,000,000 U/1.0 ML RESPECTIVELY.

a) Which concentration should you select?
b) How much sterile water should be added to the vial?
c) How much medication should be administered?
d) How should the medication be administered and how often?
e) How should the vial be relabeled?

Calculate the rate of IV flow.

32.

IV ORDER
Name: PRINCETON, MARTIN   **RM–BD:** 302–1
1,000 ML 5% D/W 8 HR

(The drop factor is 12.)

33.

IV ORDER
Name: COLE, BERNARD   **RM–BD:** 427–2
100 ML N/S 4 HR

(The drop factor is 60.)

34.

IV ORDER	
Name: MONTGOMERY, RAY	**RM–BD:** 431–C
800 ML 5% D/W 6 HR	

(The drop factor is 10.)

35.

IV ORDER	
Name: BENNETT, RHEA	**RM–BD:** 605–2
1,200 ML 5% GLUCOSE 8 HR	

(The drop factor is 15.)

36.

IV ORDER	
Name: GREENFIELD, FLO	**RM–BD:** 782–1
300 ML 10% GLUCOSE 6 HR	

(The drop factor is 60.)

Calculate the original rate of IV flow and the revised rate of flow.

37.

IV ORDER WORKSHEET

NAME: LaSalle, Albert		**RM–BD:** 109–D			
			AMT LEFT AT END OF SHIFT		
	TIME START	TIME END	0700	1500	2300
1,000 ml 5% D/W 8 hr	1800	0200		400	

(The drop factor is 12.)

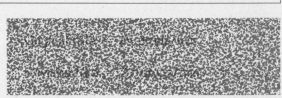

38.

IV ORDER WORKSHEET

NAME: Yale, Joyce		RM–BD: 621–A			
	TIME START	TIME END	AMT LEFT AT END OF SHIFT		
			0700	1500	2300
1,500 ml 5% glucose 12 hr	0800	2000	650		

(The drop factor is 15.)

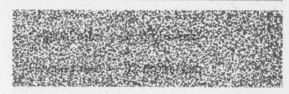

39.

IV ORDER WORKSHEET

NAME: Polk, Bennet		RM–BD: 327–4			
	TIME START	TIME END	AMT LEFT AT END OF SHIFT		
			0700	1500	2300
800 ml N/S 6 hr	1100	1700	300		

(The drop factor is 10.)

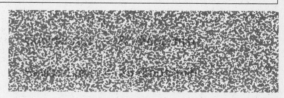

40.

IV ORDER WORKSHEET

NAME: Raleigh, Glenn		RM–BD: 101–4			
	TIME START	TIME END	AMT LEFT AT END OF SHIFT		
			0700	1500	2300
2,000 ml 5% D/W 12 hr	1030	2230	1,300		

(The drop factor is 15.)

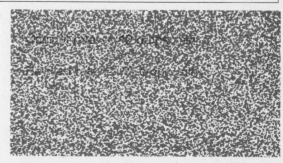

41.

IV ORDER WORKSHEET

NAME: Burton, Bradford		RM–BD: 341–4			
	TIME START	TIME END	AMT LEFT AT END OF SHIFT		
			0700	1500	2300
500 ml 5% D/W 4 hr	2100	0100		275	

(The drop factor is 15.)

42.

IV ORDER WORKSHEET

NAME: Rose, Mina		RM–BD: 706–1			
	TIME START	TIME END	AMT LEFT AT END OF SHIFT		
			0700	1500	2300
1,000 ml N/S 12 hr	0900	2100	550		

(The drop factor is 12.)

For the following orders calculate the amount of medication to be added to the IV bottle and also the rate of IV flow, assuming that the volume of IV fluid is not changed by the addition of the medication.

43.

IV ORDER		
Name: POLK, ADAM		**RM–BD:** 239–1
Solution	**Time**	**Available Medication**
1,000 ML N/S + 48 MEQ KCL	8 HR	3.2 MEQ/1.0 ML

(The drop factor is 12.)

44.

IV ORDER		
Name: HARRISON, DANNY		**RM–BD:** 921–3
Solution	**Time**	**Available Medication**
1,000 ML N/S + 17 MEQ $MgSO_4$	12 HR	81.2 MEQ/100 ML

(The drop factor is 15.)

45.

IV ORDER		
Name: HARTMAN, FRAN		**RM–BD:** 440–2
Solution	**Time**	**Available Medication**
500 ML 5% D/W + 9 MEQ CALCIUM GLUCONATE	6 HR	0.45 MEQ/1.0 ML

(The drop factor is 10.)

46.

IV ORDER		
Name: REID, BERTRAM		**RM–BD:** 223–C
Solution	**Time**	**Available Medication**
1,000 ML N/S + 20 MEQ KCL	8 HR	2 MEQ/1.0 ML

(The drop factor is 15.)

47.

IV ORDER		
Name: TRIPP, CECIL		**RM–BD:** 622–A
Solution	**Time**	**Available Medication**
1,000 ML 5% D/W + 22.3 MEQ NaHCO₃	8 HR	44.6 MEQ/50 ML

(The drop factor is 10.)

For the following orders, calculate the rate of flow of the piggybacks, and also the rate of flow between piggybacks.

48.

IV ORDER		
Name: ROCHESTER, MILDRED	**RM–BD:** 500–A	
2,000 ML 5% D/W 18 HR		

Name: ROCHESTER, MILDRED		**RM–BD:** 500–A
Medication Order	**Time**	**Available Medication**
AMPICILLIN 500 MG IVPB Q6H	30 MIN	1.0 G
Directions		
DISSOLVE IN 50 ML 5% D/W.		

(The drop factor is 12.)

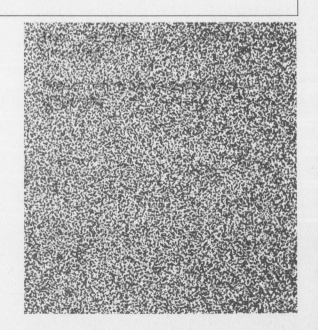

49.

IV ORDER	
Name: SANFORD, ROLF	**RM–BD:** 873–4
2,500 ML 5% GLUCOSE 24 HR	

Name: SANFORD, ROLF		**RM–BD:** 873–4
Medication Order	**Time**	**Available Medication**
500,000 U PENICILLIN IVPB Q4H	1 HR	5,000,000

Directions for Reconstitution

ADD 8.2 ML STERILE WATER. RECONSTITUTED SOLUTION WILL CONTAIN
500,000 U/1.0 ML AND MUST BE REFRIGERATED.

Directions for Piggyback

DISSOLVE IN 50 ML 5% GLUCOSE.

(This drop factor is 12.)

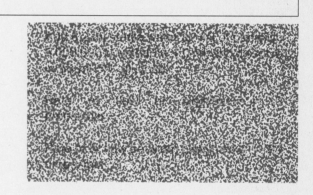

50.

IV ORDER	
Name: TOLBER, IRVING	**RM–BD:** 431–4
1,000 ML 5% D/W 12 HR	

Name: TOLBER, IRVING		**RM–BD:** 431–4
Medication Order	**Time**	**Available Medication**
KEFLIN 500 MG IVPB Q4H	1 HR	500 MG/100 ML 5% D/W

(The drop factor is 15.)

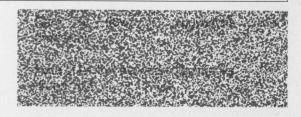

51.

IV ORDER		
Name: BERK, MAURICE		**RM–BD:** 408-2
1,000 ML N/S 8 HR		

Name: BERK, MAURICE		**RM–BD:** 408-2
Medication Order	**Time**	**Available Medication**
AMPICILLIN 500 MG IVPB Q4H	1 HR	500 MG

Directions for Reconstitution

ADD 1.8 ML STERILE WATER. RECONSTITUTED SOLUTION WILL CONTAIN 250 MG/1.0 ML.

Directions for Piggyback

DISSOLVE IN 100 ML N/S.

(The drop factor is 15.)

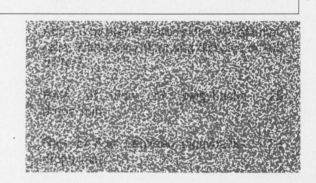

52.

IV ORDER		
Name: TURNER, JENNIE		**RM–BD:** 508-2
1,500 ML 5% D/W 12 HR		

Name: TURNER, JENNIE		**RM–BD:** 508-2
Medication Order	**Time**	**Available Medication**
CHLORAMPHENICOL 500 MG IVPB Q6H	30 MIN	500 MG/50 ML 5% D/W

(The drop factor is 12.)

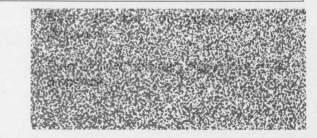

What will be the time of IV flow in the following orders?

53.

IV ORDER	
Name: FISKE, TED	**RM–BD:** 362–3
1,000 ML 5% D/W 40 DROPS/MIN	

(The drop factor is 12.)

54.

IV ORDER	
Name: GARRISON, PAULA	**RM–BD:** 406–2
125 ML N/S 25 MICRODROPS/MIN	

(The drop factor is 60.)

55.

IV ORDER	
Name: HUGHES, JOSEPH	**RM–BD:** 796–B
800 ML 5% DEXTROSE 40 DROPS/MIN	

(The drop factor is 10.)

56.

IV ORDER	
Name: ARTHUR, ROSEANNE	**RM–BD:** 1043–D
1,250 ML 5% D/W 50 DROPS/MIN	

(The drop factor is 15.)

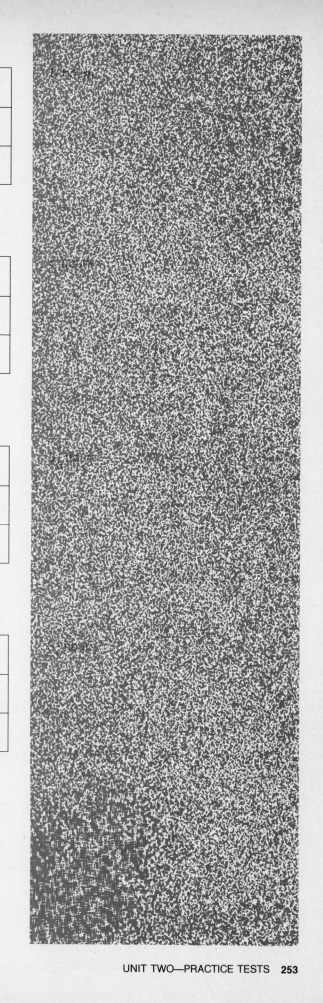

57.

IV ORDER	
Name: KARLOV, CLARKE	**RM–BD:** 668–3
900 ML 10% GLUCOSE 40 DROPS/MIN	

(The drop factor is 15.)

58.

IV ORDER	
Name: OLBERG, VIOLA	**RM–BD:** 524–A
1,500 ML 5% D/W 125 ML/HR	

59.

IV ORDER	
Name: SEARS, JOSHUA	**RM–BD:** 809–2
1,000 ML N/S 100 ML/HR	

60.

IV ORDER	
Name: SILVERS, LYNNE	**RM–BD:** 712–1
500 ML 5% GLUCOSE 75 ML/HR	

61. What will be the rate of IV flow in question #58 if the drop factor is 12?

62. What will be the rate of IV flow in question #59 if the drop factor is 10?

63. What will be the rate of IV flow in question #60 if the drop factor is 15?

64. How many milliequivalents of Fe^{2+} are present in a 300-mg ferrous sulfate tablet? Molecular weight is 278.

65. A patient was given 800 ml IV in 4 hours. This solution contained 500 ml of 5% protein hydrolysate, 200 ml of 40% glucose, and 100 ml of saline solution. How many Calories were administered?

66. A patient is to receive 4 gm of KCl daily. How many mEq potassium did he receive? Molecular weight of KCl is 75.

67. An infant is to receive 250 ml 5% glucose IV. How many Calories will the infant receive?

68. How many mEq of K^+ are present in each milliliter of a 24% potassium chloride solution? Molecular weight is 75.

69. A patient is given 1,250 ml of 10% fructose solution in 6 hours. How many Calories did he receive?

70. How many milliequivalents of Ca^{2+} are present in each milliliter of a 5% solution of calcium chloride, molecular weight 147?

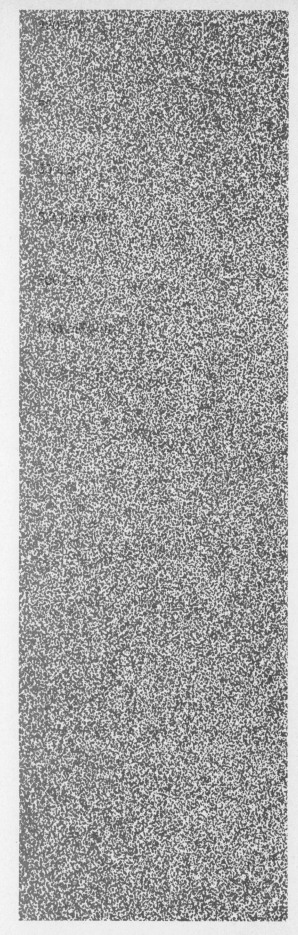

Unit Two   Practice Test No. 3

1. a) 39.8°C = _____ °F
    b) 48 kg = _____ pounds
    c) 151 cm = _____ in.
    d) 3 mcg = _____ mg
    e) 0.085 m = _____ cm

2. a) 120 kg = _____ pounds
    b) 0.004 g = _____ mg
    c) 20 ml = _____ cc
    d) 2 tsp = _____ ml
    e) 10 drops = _____ ml

3. a) 2 mcg = _____ mg
    b) 0.04 g = _____ mg
    c) 25 cm = _____ m
    d) 100°F = _____ °C
    e) 5'8" = _____ cm

4. A patient's weight, temperature, and height were re-corded as 175 pounds, 102.4°F, and 6'2". Convert these figures to a) kg, b) °C, and c) cm.

For questions 5–9 calculate the number of tablets or cap-sules to be administered.

5.

Name: WEXLER, VIOLA	**RM–BD:** 105–4
Medication Order	**Available Medication**
DIGOXIN 0.5 MG	TABLETS 250 MCG

6.

Name: NOVELLO, SHELDON	**RM–BD:** 809–C
Medication Order	**Available Medication**
PREMARIN 625 MCG	TABLETS 0.625 MG

7.

Name: SPORN, PENNY	**RM–BD:** 503–B
Medication Order	**Available Medication**
TETRACYCLINE 0.25 G	CAPSULES 250 MG

8.

Name: SUDBURY, LILLY	RM–BD: 562–C
Medication Order	**Available Medication**
LOXITANE 0.02 G	CAPSULES 10 MG

9.

Name: FOOTE, ANDREA	RM–BD: 404–2
Medication Order	**Available Medication**
SYNTHROID 0.3 MG	TABLETS 150 MCG

Write statements for the following orders.

10.

Name: BURNS, DOREEN	RM–BD: 227–1
Medication Order	**Available Medication**
MORPHINE SULFATE 10 MG SUBQ PRN	15 MG/1.0 ML

11.

Name: SCOTT, BLANCHE	RM–BD: 302–A
Medication Order	**Available Medication**
SODIUM AMPICILLIN 750 MG IM Q6H	1 G

Directions for reconstitution

ADD 2.4 ML STERILE WATER.
RECONSTITUTED LIQUID WILL CONTAIN 400
MG/1.0 ML AND MUST BE USED WITHIN 1
HOUR.

12.

Name: SINCLAIR, RUSSELL	**RM–BD:** 305–D
Wt. in kg. 20.0	

Medication Order	**Available Medication**
KANTREX IM Q6H	75 MG/2 ML

Pediatric Dosage
15 MG/KG/DAY

13.

Name: ALVAREZ, JUANITA	**RM–BD:** 303–A

Medication Order	**Available Medication**
MAGNESIUM SULFATE 40 G HS	50%

14.

Name: TRASK, SYDNEY	**RM–BD:** 239–1
Wt. in kg. 10.0	

Medication Order	**Available Medication**
VELOSEF Q12H	250 MG/5 ML

Pediatric Dosage
25 MG/KG/DAY

15.

Name: KEYSTONE, ANGELA	**RM–BD:** 405–1

Medication Order	**Available Medication**
TICARCILLIN SODIUM 0.6 G IM TID	3G

Directions for reconstitution

ADD 6 ML STERILE WATER. RECONSTITUTED
SOLUTION WILL CONTAIN 1 G/2.5 ML AND
IS STABLE FOR 24 HOURS AT ROOM
TEMPERATURE AND FOR 72 HOURS IF
REFRIGERATED.

16.

Name: GREENWOOD, LOUIS	**RM–BD:** 203–4

Medication Order	**Available Medication**
EPINEPHRINE 100 MCG SUBQ STAT	1:1,1000

17.

Name: COLLINS, JONI	**RM–BD:** 431–A
Wt. in kg. 32.0	

Medication Order	**Available Medication**
ERYTHROMYCIN SULFATE QID	400 MG/5 ML

Pediatric Dosage

50 MG/KG/DAY

18.

Name: TRIPP, BECKY	**RM–BD:** 163–2

Medication Order	**Available Medication**
KCL 6.7 MEQ QAM	20 MEQ/15 ML

19.

Name: NORTON, MERV	**RM–BD:** 606–2

Medication Order	**Available Medication**
PENICILLIN G 200,000 U IM QID	1,000,000 U

Directions for reconstitution

ADD 9.6 ML, 4.6 ML, OR 3.6 ML STERILE
DILUENT TO PROVIDE 100,000 U/1.0 ML,
200,000 U/1.0 ML, OR 250,000 U/1.0 ML
RESPECTIVELY.

a) Which concentration should you select?
b) How much diluent should be added to the vial?
c) How much reconstituted penicillin G should be withdrawn?
d) How should the medication be administered and how often?
e) How should the vial be relabeled?
f) How many doses are possible from that vial?

20.

Name: DAYSTROM, JAMES	**RM–BD:** 704–1
Wt. in kg. 20.0	

Medication Order	**Available Medication**
TETRACYCLINE HYDROCHLORIDE Q6H	125 MG/5 ML

Pediatric Dosage

25 MG/KG/DAY

21.

Name: KELLER, RENE	**RM–BD:** 203–D

Medication Order	**Available Medication**
VITAMIN B$_{12}$ 500 MCG IM QD	1,000 MCG/1.0 ML

22.

Name: SPRING, ROCKY	RM–BD: 403–2
Medication Order	**Available Medication**
CHLORPROMAZINE 25 MG IM BID	50 MG/2 ML

23.

Name: KENNICOTT, ARTHUR	RM–BD: 193–A
Medication Order	**Available Medication**
STREPTOMYCIN 0.4 G IM BID	5 G

Directions for reconstitution

ADD 6.5 ML STERILE WATER. RECONSTITUTED SOLUTION WILL CONTAIN 500 MG/1.0 ML. STORE IN REFRIGERATOR FOR NOT MORE THAN 14 DAYS.

24.

Name: ALLEN, JOYCE	RM–BD: 652–3
Medication Order	**Available Medication**
PENICILLIN G 500,000 U IM QID	5,000,000 U

Directions for reconstitution

ADD 23 ML, 18 ML, 8 ML, OR 3 ML STERILE DILUENT TO PROVIDE 200,000 U/1.0 ML, 250,000 U/1.0 ML, 500,000 U/1.0 ML, OR 1,000,000 U/1.0 ML RESPECTIVELY.

25.

Name: BERGEN, TONI	RM–BD: 332–1
Medication Order	**Available Medication**
COMPAZINE 5 MG IM Q4H	10 MG/2 ML

26.

Name: FLYNN, GREGORY	RM–BD: 125–4
Medication Order	**Available Medication**
INSULIN 20 U SUBQ QAM (USE A TUBERCULIN SYRINGE)	100 U/1.0 ML

27.

Name: BERWYN, PAUL	RM–BD: 119–4
Medication Order	**Available Medication**
TOFRANIL 12.5 MG IM QID	25 MG/2 CC

28.

Name: BOGAN, VINCENT	RM–BD: 230–A
Medication Order	**Available Medication**
PENICILLIN G 200,000 U IM Q4H	1,000,000 U

Directions for reconstitution

ADD 9.6 ML STERILE WATER. RECONSTITUTED SOLUTION WILL CONTAIN 200,000 U/1.0 ML.

29.

Name: BERNARD, LEO	RM–BD: 346–2
Medication Order	**Available Medication**
THIAMINE 0.05 G IM QD	100 MG/1.0 ML

30.

Name: STANLEY, ROGER	**RM–BD:** 451–C

Medication Order	**Available Medication**
AMPICILLIN TRIHYDRATE 750 MG QID	5.0 G

Directions for reconstitution

ADD 70 ML WATER. RECONSTITUTED SOLUTION WILL CONTAIN 250 MG/5 ML AND IS STABLE FOR 14 DAYS WHEN REFRIGERATED.

31.

Name: MOELLER, ROY	**RM–BD:** 239–B

Medication Order	**Available Medication**
ELAVIL 20 MG IM TID	10 MG/1.0 ML

Calculate the rate of IV flow for questions 32–36.

32.

IV ORDER	
Name: BARON, BONNIE	**RM–BD:** 506–3
800 ML 5% D/W 6 HR	

(The drop factor is 10.)

33.

IV ORDER	
Name: WOLPERT, VERA	**RM–BD:** 532–A
2,000 ML 5% D/W 24 HR	

(The drop factor is 12.)

34.

IV ORDER
Name: EUCLID, IDA   **RM–BD:** 403–2
1,200 ML N/S   12 HR

(The drop factor is 15.)

35.

IV ORDER
Name: TUFTS, GRACE   **RM–BD:** 761–4
500 ML 10% GLUCOSE   10 HR

(The drop factor is 60.)

36.

IV ORDER
Name: YATES, APRIL   **RM–BD:** 305–2
100 ML 5% D/W   4 HR

(The drop factor is 60.)

Calculate the original rate of IV flow and the revised rate of flow for questions 37–41.

37.

IV ORDER WORKSHEET

NAME: Karster, Toni **RM–BD:** 109–2					
			AMT LEFT AT END OF SHIFT		
	TIME START	TIME END	0700	1500	2300
1,000 ml 5% D/W 8 hr	0800	1600	150		

(The drop factor is 12.)

38.

IV ORDER WORKSHEET

NAME: Briggs, Earl	RM–BD: 375–A				
			AMT LEFT AT END OF SHIFT		
	TIME START	TIME END	0700	1500	2300
1,500 ml N/S 12 hr	1200	2400	1150		

(The drop factor is 10.)

39.

IV ORDER WORKSHEET

NAME: Croft, Carol	RM–BD: 457–D				
			AMT LEFT AT END OF SHIFT		
	TIME START	TIME END	0700	1500	2300
750 ml 10% glucose 6 hr	2100	0300		550	

(The drop factor is 15.)

40.

IV ORDER WORKSHEET

NAME: Waxman, Edna	RM–BD: 506–B				
			AMT LEFT AT END OF SHIFT		
	TIME START	TIME END	0700	1500	2300
2,000 ml 5% D/W 12 hr	1800	0600		1600	

(The drop factor is 12.)

41.

IV ORDER WORKSHEET

NAME: Parker, Sarah		RM–BD: 803–1			
				AMT LEFT AT END OF SHIFT	
	TIME START	TIME END	0700	1500	2300
500 ml N/S 4 hr	1400	1800	400		

(The drop factor is 15.)

For the following orders calculate the rate of flow of the piggybacks, and also the rate of flow between piggybacks.

42.

IV ORDER
Name: ROADSTONE, DON   RM–BD: 462–1
2,000 ML 5% D/W 24 HR

Name: ROADSTONE, DON		RM–BD: 462–1
Medication Order	**Time**	**Available Medication**
AMPICILLIN 500 MG IVPB	1 HR	1 G

Directions for Reconstitution

ADD 3.5 ML STERILE WATER. RECONSTITUTED SOLUTION WILL CONTAIN 250 MG/1.0 ML.

Directions for Piggyback

DISSOLVE IN 100 ML 5% D/W.

(The drop factor is 12.)

43.

IV ORDER	
Name: CORDAY, DELLA	**RM–BD:** 502–C
2,000 ML N/S 24 HR	

Name: CORDAY, DELLA		**RM–BD:** 502–C
Medication Order	**Time**	**Available Medication**
KEFLIN 500 MG IVPB Q4H	30 MIN	500 MG/100 ML N/S

(The drop factor is 12.)

44.

IV ORDER	
Name: TRIPP, DONNA	**RM–BD:** 721–D
2,000 ML 5% D/W 16 HR	

Name: TRIPP, DONNA		**RM–BD:** 721–D
Medication Order	**Time**	**Available Medication**
PENICILLIN G 500,000 U IVPB Q4H	1 HR	5,000,000 U

Directions for Reconstitution

ADD 8.0 ML STERILE WATER TO PROVIDE 500,000 U/1.0 ML.

Directions for Piggyback

DISSOLVE IN 100 ML 5% D/W.

(The drop factor is 10.)

45.

IV ORDER		
Name: HUXTON, GILBERT	**RM–BD:** 1812–2	
2,500 ML N/S 24 HR		

Name: HUXTON, GILBERT		**RM–BD:** 1812–2
Medication Order	**Time**	**Available Medication**
CHLORAMPHENICOL 500 MG IVPB Q6H	1 HR	500 MG/50 ML N/S

(The drop factor is 10.)

46.

IV ORDER		
Name: DUNNE, NANCY	**RM–BD:** 602–A	
1,500 ML N/S 18 HR		

Name: DUNNE, NANCY		**RM–BD:** 602–A
Medication Order	**Time**	**Available Medication**
SODIUM METHICILLIN 1 G IVPB Q6H	1 HR	1 G
Directions		
DISSOLVE IN 50 ML N/S.		

(The drop factor is 12.)

For the following orders calculate the amount of medication to be added to the IV bottle and also the rate of IV flow, assuming that the volume of IV fluid is not changed by the addition of the medication.

47.

```
                     IV ORDER

Name: SIMS, ELIZABETH         RM-BD: 805-A

Solution              Time    Available Medication

1,000 ML N/S          8 HR    2 MEQ/1.0 ML
+ 10 MEQ KCL
```

(The drop factor is 12.)

48.

```
                     IV ORDER

Name: CLAY, KAREN             RM-BD: 157-C

Solution              Time    Available Medication

500 ML 5% D/W         4 HR    0.9 MEQ/1.0 ML
+ 4.5 MEQ
CALCIUM
GLUCONATE
```

(The drop factor is 15.)

49.

```
                     IV ORDER

Name: NORDELL, KIM            RM-BD: 301-D

Solution              Time    Available Medication

1,000 ML N/S          8 HR    44.6 MEQ/50 ML
+ 9 MEQ SODIUM
BICARBONATE
```

(The drop factor is 12.)

50.

```
                    IV ORDER

Name: HOBART, DEREK            RM–BD: 982–3


Solution                Time    Available Medication

1,000 ML 5% D/W         8 HR    1.36 MEQ/1.0 ML
+ 1 MEQ CALCIUM
CHLORIDE
```

(The drop factor is 15.)

51.

```
                    IV ORDER

Name: PORTER, CARRIE           RM–BD: 772–1


Solution                Time    Available Medication

500 ML N/S +            4 HR    81.2 MEQ/100 ML
6 MEQ MAGNESIUM
SULFATE
```

(The drop factor is 10.)

How long will the IV flow in the following orders?

52.

```
                    IV ORDER

Name: LAMB, BAXTER             RM–BD: 702–2


1,000 ML N/S   50 DROPS/MIN
```

(The drop factor is 15.)

53.

```
                    IV ORDER

Name: MENDICOTT, LAURA         RM–BD: 803–1


150 ML 10% GLUCOSE   30 MICRODROPS/MIN
```

(The drop factor is 60.)

54.

IV ORDER	
Name: NEWTON, OLIVER	**RM–BD:** 152–C
1,200 ML 5% D/W 40 DROPS/MIN	

(The drop factor is 10.)

55.

IV ORDER	
Name: HARDY, ALICE	**RM–BD:** 203–D
200 ML 10% DEXTROSE 25 MICRODROPS/MIN	

(The drop factor is 60.)

56.

IV ORDER	
Name: TORRANCE, JEFFREY	**RM–BD:** 375–2
2,500 ML N/S 17 DROPS/MIN	

(The drop factor is 12.)

57.

IV ORDER	
Name: WELLER, MARCUS	**RM–BD:** 418–4
1,000 ML 5% D/W 83 ML/HR	

58.

IV ORDER	
Name: BASHWELL, TANYA	**RM–BD:** 118–3
125 ML N/S 25 ML/HR	

59.

IV ORDER
Name: HENRY, SYLVIA   **RM–BD:** 330–1
1,200 ML 5% D/W   150 ML/HR

60. What will be the rate of IV flow in question #57 if the drop factor is 15?

61. What will be the rate of IV flow in question #58 if the drop factor is 60?

62. What will be the rate of IV flow in question #59 if the drop factor is 12?

63. How many mEq/ml of Na^+ are in a 10% solution of sodium chloride, molecular weight 58.5?

64. An infant is given 100 ml IV in 4 hours. The solution contains 60 ml of 6% protein hydrolysate, 30 ml of 50% glucose, and 10 ml of saline solution. How many Calories were administered? What should be the rate of flow for the IV? The drop factor is 60.

65. How many milliequivalents of Ca^{2+} are present in 200 mg calcium lactate, molecular weight 308?

66. An infant was given 100 ml of 6% dextran (a carbohydrate) IV in 3 hours. How many Calories did she recieve? What should be the rate of administering the IV? The drop factor is 60.

67. How many mEq/ml of Mg^{2+} are in a 10% solution of magnesium sulfate, molecular weight 244?

68. A patient is given 1,500 ml IV in 12 hours. The solution contains 800 ml of 6% protein hydrolysate, 600 ml of 40% glucose solution, and 100 ml of saline solution. How many Calories were administered? What should be the rate of administration if the drop factor is 15?

69. How many milliequivalents of Ca^{2+} are present in each milliliter of a 1% solution of calcium levulinate, molecular weight 288?

70. An infant was given 150 ml of 5% dextran IV. How many Calories did she receive?

Unit Two   Practice Test No. 4

1. a) 36.8°C = _____ °F
   b) 0.05 mg = _____ mcg
   c) 1 tablespoonful = _____ ml
   d) 110 pounds = _____ kg
   e) 5'8" = _____ cm

2. a) 0.25 ml = _____ drops
   b) 0.05 liters = _____ ml
   c) 100 mcg = _____ mg
   d) 1 teaspoonful = _____ ml
   e) 124 cm = _____ in.

3. a) 75 kg = _____ lb
   b) 100.6°F = _____ °C
   c) 0.4% of 500 ml = _____ ml
   d) 37.5 cm = _____ m
   e) 37.5 m = _____ km

4. A patient's weight, temperature, and height were re-corded as 60.4 kg, 38.8°C, and 178 cm. Convert these figures to a) pounds, b) °F, and c) inches.

For questions 5–9 calculate the number of tablets or cap-sules to be administered.

5.

Name: FORDHAM, BETTE	**RM–BD:** 330–1
Medication Order	**Available Medication**
ALLOPURINOL 0.15 G	TABLETS 300 MG

6.

Name: MANOPOULOS, TED	**RM–BD:** 305–2
Medication Order	**Available Medication**
CHLOROTHIAZIDE 0.5 MG	TABLETS 250 MCG

7.

Name: HART, BERNICE	**RM–BD:** 652–3
Medication Order	**Available Medication**
ERYTHROMYCIN 250 MG	TABLETS 0.25 G

8.

Name: FOREST, BURTON	RM–BD: 321–1
Medication Order	**Available Medication**
TETRACYCLINE 500 MG	CAPSULES 250 MG

9.

Name: ROSE, KEITH	RM–BD: 431–4
Medication Order	**Available Medication**
TERRAMYCIN 250 MG	CAPSULES 0.25 G

Write statements for the following orders.

10.

Name: FOX, JOEL	RM–BD: 456–3
Medication Order	**Available Medication**
MORPHINE SULFATE 5 MG SUBQ PRN	15 MG/1.0 ML

11.

Name: KEYSTONE, ANGELA	RM–BD: 903–4
Medication Order	**Available Medication**
PENICILLIN G 500,000 U IM QID	5,000,000 U

Directions for Reconstitution

ADD 18 ML STERILE WATER. RECONSTITUTED SOLUTION WILL CONTAIN 250,000 U/1.0 ML AND IS STABLE FOR 1 WEEK IF REFRIGERATED.

12.

Name: SWIFT, NORMA	**RM–BD:** 348–2
Wt. in kg. 20.0	

Medication Order	**Available Medication**
VELOSEF Q12H	250 MG/5 ML

Pediatric Dosage
25 MG/KG/DAY

13.

Name: SLOAT, ROBERTA	**RM–BD:** 372–A

Medication Order	**Available Medication**
PROCHLORPERAZINE 5 MG IM Q4H	10 MG/2 CC

14.

Name: MCLEOD, KEVIN	**RM–BD:** 404–1

Medication Order	**Available Medication**
AMPICILLIN TRIHYDRATE 500 MG QID	5.0 G

Directions for Reconstitution
ADD 70 ML WATER. RECONSTITUTED SOLUTION WILL CONTAIN 250 MG/5 ML AND IS STABLE FOR 14 DAYS WHEN REFRIGERATED.

15.

Name: HOLT, MARIBETH	**RM–BD:** 164–D
Wt. in kg. 5.0	

Medication Order	Available Medication
KANAMYCIN IM BID	75 MG/2 ML

Pediatric Dosage
15 MG/KG/DAY

16.

Name: SANDERS, GARY	**RM–BD:** 338–3

Medication Order	Available Medication
PENICILLIN G 500,000 U IM QID	5,000,000 U

Directions for Reconstitution

ADD 8 ML STERILE WATER. RECONSTITUTED SOLUTION WILL CONTAIN 500,000 U/1.0 ML AND IS STABLE FOR 1 WEEK WHEN REFRIGERATED.

17.

Name: NORTON, MERV	**RM–BD:** 339–A

Medication Order	Available Medication
KCL 20 MEQ BID	40 MEQ/15 ML

18.

Name: ALLEN, JOYCE	**RM–BD:** 208–4

Medication Order	**Available Medication**
SODIUM AMPICILLIN 500 MG IM TID	1 G

Directions for Reconstitution

ADD 3.5 ML STERILE WATER. RECONSTITUTED SOLUTION WILL CONTAIN 250 MG/1.0 ML AND MUST BE USED WITHIN 1 HOUR.

19.

Name: BENDER, NORA	**RM–BD:** 223–B
Wt. in kg. 30.0	

Medication Order	**Available Medication**
OMNIPEN Q8H	125 MG/5 ML

Pediatric Dosage

25 MG/KG/DAY

20.

Name: CLARK, STEVE	**RM–BD:** 742–A

Medication Order	**Available Medication**
INSULIN 70 U SUBQ QAM (USE TUBERCULIN SYRINGE)	100 U/1.0 ML

21.

Name: WOOD, MICHAEL	**RM–BD:** 506–C

Medication Order	**Available Medication**
TICARCILLIN SODIUM 0.5 G IM TID	3 G

Directions for reconstitution

ADD 6 ML STERILE WATER. RECONSTITUTED
SOLUTION WILL CONTAIN 1 G/2.5 ML AND
IS STABLE FOR 24 HOURS AT ROOM
TEMPERATURE AND FOR 72 HOURS IF
REFRIGERATED.

22.

Name: ANDRE, HOWARD	**RM–BD:** 203–4

Medication Order	**Available Medication**
LANOXIN 0.25 MG IM Q6H	500 MCG/2 CC

23.

Name: SCHMIDT, HANS	**RM–BD:** 109–2

Medication Order	**Available Medication**
EPINEPHRINE 750 MCG SUBQ STAT	1:1,000

24.

Name: TOWLE, CONSTANCE	**RM–BD:** 378–2

Medication Order	**Available Medication**
SODIUM AMPICILLIN 375 MG IM Q6H	1 G

Directions for reconstitution

ADD 2.4 ML STERILE WATER.
RECONSTITUTED SOLUTION WILL CONTAIN
400 MG/1.0 ML AND MUST BE USED WITHIN
1 HOUR.

25.

Name: BRADLEY, ERNEST	**RM–BD:** 393–B
Wt. in kg. 4.0	

Medication Order	**Available Medication**
GARAMYCIN IM Q8H	10 MG/1.0 ML

Pediatric Dosage
7.5 MG/KG/DAY

26.

Name: REID, FRANK	**RM–BD:** 451–D

Medication Order	**Available Medication**
STREPTOMYCIN 0.5 G IM BID	5 G

Directions for reconstitution
ADD 6.5 ML STERILE WATER. RECONSTITUTED SOLUTION WILL CONTAIN 500 MG/1.0 ML. STORE IN REFRIGERATOR FOR NOT MORE THAN 14 DAYS.

27.

Name: NORDHOFF, CLARENCE	**RM–BD:** 532–C

Medication Order	**Available Medication**
KCL 10 MEQ QID	40 MEQ/30 ML

28.

Name: GRAYSON, KIM	**RM–BD:** 802–A

Medication Order	**Available Medication**
VITAMIN B_{12} 0.75 MG IM QD	1,000 MCG/1.0 ML

29.

Name: GREEN, VIRGINIA	RM–BD: 902–1

Medication Order	Available Medication
PENICILLIN G 200,000 U IM QID	5,000,000 U

Directions for reconstitution

ADD 23 ML, 18 ML, 8 ML, OR 3 ML
STERILE DILUENT TO PROVIDE 200,000
U/1.0 ML, 250,000 U/1.0 ML, 500,000
U/1.0 ML, OR 1,000,000 U/1.0 ML
RESPECTIVELY.

  a) What concentration should you select?
  b) How much sterile water should be added to the vial?
  c) How much medication should be administered?
  d) How should the medication be administered and how often?
  e) How should the vial be relabeled?
  f) How many doses are possible from the vial?

30.

Name: HINKLEY, LILA	RM–BD: 1014–A

Medication Order	Available Medication
MAGNESIUM SULFATE 25 G HS	50%

31.

Name: RAVENSWOOD, DIANE	RM–BD: 267–C

Medication Order	Available Medication
THIAMINE 50 MG IM QD	0.1 G/1.0 ML

Calculate the rate of IV flow for questions 32–37.

32.

IV ORDER	
Name: SIMON, MELVIN	**RM–BD:** 548–2
1,000 ML 5% D/W 8 HR	

(The drop factor is 15.)

33.

IV ORDER	
Name: FRENCH, HILARY	**RM–BD:** 607–4
120 ML 10% GLUCOSE 6 HR	

(The drop factor is 60.)

34.

IV ORDER	
Name: HUNTER, HAROLD	**RM–BD:** 123–2
2,000 ML N/S 24 HR	

(The drop factor is 10.)

35.

IV ORDER	
Name: SHERRY, BRIAN	**RM–BD:** 316–A
800 ML 5% D/W 6 HR	

(The drop factor is 12.)

36.

IV ORDER	
Name: DALLAS, TRICIA	**RM–BD:** 541–3
900 ML 5% GLUCOSE 8 HR	

(The drop factor is 15.)

37.

IV ORDER	
Name: FOX, CARL	**RM–BD:** 629–D
300 ML 10% GLUCOSE 12 HR	

(The drop factor is 60.)

Calculate the original rate of IV flow and also the revised rate of IV flow at the beginning of the next shift.

38.

IV ORDER WORKSHEET

NAME: Carter, Kenneth		RM–BD: 870–2	AMT LEFT AT END OF SHIFT		
	TIME START	TIME END	0700	1500	2300
1,000 5% D/W 8 hr	2200	0600		900	

(The drop factor is 10.)

39.

IV ORDER WORKSHEET

NAME: Kostner, Tess		RM–BD: 1022–4	AMT LEFT AT END OF SHIFT		
	TIME START	TIME END	0700	1500	2300
1,500 ml N/S 12 hr	1600	0400		700	

(The drop factor is 10.)

40.

IV ORDER WORKSHEET

NAME: Kirk, Chris	RM–BD: 714–3				
			AMT LEFT AT END OF SHIFT		
	TIME START	TIME END	0700	1500	2300
900 ml N/S 6 hr	1900	0100		350	

(The drop factor is 12.)

41.

IV ORDER WORKSHEET

NAME: Lamon, Julia	RM–BD: 980–4				
			AMT LEFT AT END OF SHIFT		
	TIME START	TIME END	0700	1500	2300
2,000 ml 5% D/W 12 hr	1700	0500		1100	

(The drop factor is 12.)

42.

IV ORDER WORKSHEET

NAME: Dorchester, Diana	RM–BD: 508–4				
			AMT LEFT AT END OF SHIFT		
	TIME START	TIME END	0700	1500	2300
500 ml N/S 4 hr	1400	1800	400		

(The drop factor is 10.)

For the following orders calculate the amount of medication to be added to the IV bottle and also the rate of IV flow, assuming that the volume of IV fluid is not changed by the addition of the medication.

43.

IV ORDER		
Name: CONROY, LEE		**RM–BD:** 525–1
Solution	**Time**	**Available Medication**
1,000 ML N/S + 18 MEQ CALCIUM GLUCONATE	8 HR	0.45 MEQ/1.0 ML

(The drop factor is 15.)

44.

IV ORDER		
Name: MINOR, HERBERT		**RM–BD:** 830–4
Solution	**Time**	**Available Medication**
1,000 ML 5% D/W + 40 MEQ KCL	8 HR	2 MEQ/1.0 ML

(The drop factor is 12.)

45.

IV ORDER		
Name: RAYE, BARBARA		**RM–BD:** 706–1
Solution	**Time**	**Available Medication**
500 ML N/S + 8.5 MEQ $MgSO_4$	4 HR	81.2 MEQ/100 ML

(The drop factor is 10.)

46.

IV ORDER		
Name: MENARD, WAYNE		**RM–BD:** 1002–3
Solution	**Time**	**Available Medication**
1,000 ML N/S + 1 MEQ CALCIUM CHLORIDE	8 HR	1.36 MEQ/1.0 ML

(The drop factor is 15.)

47.

IV ORDER		
Name: WASSELL, BRUNO		**RM–BD:** 100–1
Solution	**Time**	**Available Medication**
500 ML N/S + 9 MEQ CALCIUM GLUCEPTATE	4 HR	0.9 MEQ/1.0 ML

(The drop factor is 12.)

For the following orders calculate the rate of flow of the piggybacks, and also the rate of flow between piggybacks.

48.

IV ORDER	
Name: ROBINSON, LEE	**RM–BD:** 482–1
2,000 ML N/S 12 HR	

Name: ROBINSON, LEE		**RM–BD:** 482–1
Medication Order	**Time**	**Available Medication**
SODIUM METHICILLIN 1 G IVPB Q6H	1 HR	1 G

Directions for Reconstitution

ADD 1.5 ML STERILE WATER. RECONSTITUTED SOLUTION WILL CONTAIN 500 MG/1.0 ML.

Directions for Piggyback

DISSOLVE IN 50 ML N/S.

(The drop factor is 12.)

49.

IV ORDER	
Name: ALFORD, PATTY	**RM–BD:** 128–3
2,000 ML 5% D/W 24 HR	

Name: ALFORD, PATTY		**RM–BD:** 128–3
Medication Order	**Time**	**Available Medication**
CHLORAMPHENICOL 500 MG IVPB Q6H	30 MIN	500 MG/50 ML 5% D/W

(The drop factor is 12.)

50.

IV ORDER	
Name: SEDGWICK, GWEN	**RM–BD:** 329–4
2,500 ML N/S 24 HR	

Name: SEDGWICK, GWEN		**RM–BD:** 329–4
Medication Order	**Time**	**Available Medication**
KEFLIN 500 MG IVPB Q6H	20 MIN	1 G

Directions for Reconstitution

ADD 5.0 ML STERILE WATER. RECONSTITUTED SOLUTION WILL CONTAIN 200 MG/1.0 ML.

Directions for Piggyback

DISSOLVE IN 50 ML N/S.

(The drop factor is 15.)

51.

IV ORDER	
Name: DEAN, ARTHUR	**RM–BD:** 430–4
2,500 ML N/S 24 HR	

Name: DEAN, ARTHUR		**RM–BD:** 430–4
Medication Order	**Time**	**Available Medication**
AMPICILLIN 500 MG IVPB Q6H	30 MIN	1 G

Directions

DISSOLVE IN 100 ML N/S.

(The drop factor is 10.)

52.

IV ORDER		
Name: HASKELL, ANGELA	**RM–BD:** 302–4	
1,500 ML 5% D/W 18 HR		

Name: HASKELL, ANGELA		**RM–BD:** 302–4
Medication Order	**Time**	**Available Medication**
PENICILLIN G 1,000,000 U IVPB Q4H	30 MIN	1,000,000 U/100 ML 5% D/W

(The drop factor is 10.)

How long will the IV flow in the following orders?

53.

IV ORDER	
Name: MOSS, LEONA	**RM–BD:** 636–C
2,000 ML 5% D/W 40 DROPS/MIN	

(The drop factor is 12.)

54.

IV ORDER	
Name: PAUL, LEONARD	**RM–BD:** 198–D
125 ML N/S 50 MICRODROPS/MIN	

(The drop factor is 60.)

55.

IV ORDER	
Name: EDWARDS, MELVINA	**RM–BD:** 230–A
1,600 ML 5% GLUCOSE 50 DROPS/MIN	

(The drop factor is 15.)

56.

IV ORDER	
Name: VINELAND, NORTON	**RM–BD:** 402–1
100 ML 5% D/W 44 MICRODROPS/MIN	

(The drop factor is 60.)

57.

IV ORDER	
Name: SINGER, MICHELE	**RM–BD:** 651–4
2,000 ML 5% D/W 25 DROPS/MIN	

(The drop factor is 12.)

58.

IV ORDER	
Name: CARSTEN, BRYANT	**RM–BD:** 150–D
2,000 ML 5% D/W 125 ML/HR	

59.

IV ORDER	
Name: MICHAELS, BELLE	**RM–BD:** 200–1
100 ML N/S 25 ML/HR	

60.

IV ORDER	
Name: THATCHER, VERNON	**RM–BD:** 302–3
1,000 ML 5% GLUCOSE 100 ML/HR	

61. What will be the rate of IV flow in question #58 if the drop factor is 15?

62. What will be the rate of IV flow in question #59 if the drop factor is 60?

63. What will be the rate of IV flow in question #60 if the drop factor is 10?

64. How many milliequivalents of Ca^{2+} are present in a 10% calcium levulinate solution? Molecular weight is 288.

65. A patient was given 1,500 ml of solution IV in 8 hours. The solution contained 900 ml of 6% protein hydrolysate, 400 ml of 50% glucose solution, and 200 ml of saline solution. How many Calories did the patient receive? If the drop factor is 12, what should be the rate of administration?

66. A patient is to receive 300 mg calcium lactate. How many mEq of Ca^{2+} will she receive? Molecular weight is 308.

67. An infant is to receive 120 ml IV in 4 hours. The solution contains 60 ml of 5% protein hydrolysate, 40 ml of 40% glucose solution, and 20 ml of saline solution. How many Calories will the infant receive? What should be the rate of administration for the infant? Assume a drop factor of 60.

68. How many milliequivalents Ca^{2+} are present in a 250-mg tablet of calcium carbonate, molecular weight 100?

69. An infant was given 90 ml of 5% dextran (a carbohydrate) in 4 hours. How many Calories did he receive? What should be the rate of administration for the infant? The drop factor is 60.

70. How many mEq/ml Na^+ are present in a 5% solution of sodium bicarbonate, molecular weight 84?

Appendix I

Roman Numerals

Section 1   Learning to Read Roman Numerals

Look at the Roman numeral below:

i

i means 1.

Look at the following Roman numeral:

ii

ii means 2.

Whenever a Roman numeral is repeated, add the numerals. For instance:

ii = 1 + 1 = 2

1. What does iii mean?

Remember that when Roman numerals are repeated, they should be added.

Note: The Roman numeral i is always written with a dot over it.

Look at the Roman numeral below:

v

v means 5.

What does each of the following Roman numerals mean?

2. vii

3. viii

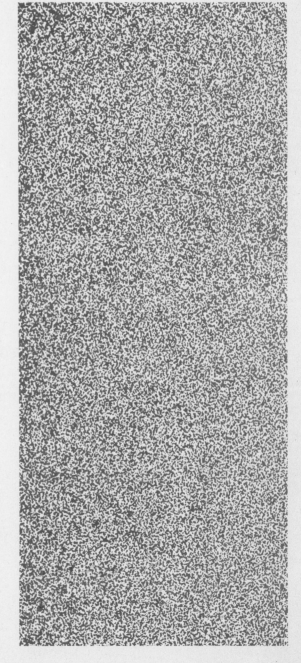

Look at the following Roman numeral:

x

x means 10.

Look at the following Roman numeral:

xx

xx means 20.

Remember that when Roman numerals are repeated, they should be added.

What does each of the following Roman numerals mean?

4. xxx

5. xxi

6. vi

7. xi

8. xv

9. xxv

10. xii

Look at the following Roman numerals:

l

c

l means 50. c means 100.

What does each of the following Roman numerals mean?

11. lv

12. cv

13. liii

14. cii

15. lx

16. cx

17. clxv

18. cxi

Passing score is no more than *3* errors.

Section 2 Learning to Read Roman Numerals (cont.)

Look at the following Roman numeral:

vi

Bear in mind that i is smaller than v. Whenever a smaller numeral follows, the numerals are added. Therefore,

vi = 5 + 1 = 6

However, look at the following Roman numeral.

iv

In this case, the smaller Roman numeral i appears before the larger numeral v. Whenever a smaller numeral appears before a larger numeral, the smaller numeral is subtracted. Therefore,

iv = 5 − 1 = 4

What does each of the following Roman numerals mean?

1. vii

2. li

3. iv

4. xc

5. ci

6. xl

7. ix

8. lii

9. lx

10. xxv

Look at the following Roman numeral:

xiv

In this case, a smaller numeral—i—appears between two larger numerals.

When a smaller numeral appears between two larger numerals, the smaller numeral is subtracted from the following numeral.

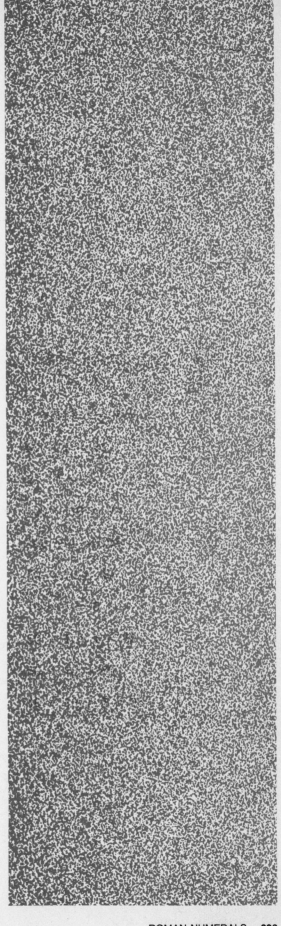

Therefore, xiv means $10 + 5 - 1 = 14$.

What does each of the following Roman numerals mean?

11. cxl

12. xiv

13. xix

14. lix

15. cxix

16. cxc

Sometimes, Roman numerals are written as capital letters.

What does each of the following Roman numerals mean?

17. XV

18. LIX

19. CXL

20. LXXVIII

21. CCX

22. LXXIX

23. XIV

24. XXXIX

25. XVIII

Section 3 How to Write Roman Numerals

Here's a helpful hint for writing Roman numerals accurately.

Consider the following number:

27

You will find it easier to break up the number into various units before changing to Roman numerals.

For instance:

$$27 = 20 + 7$$
$$27 = xxvii$$

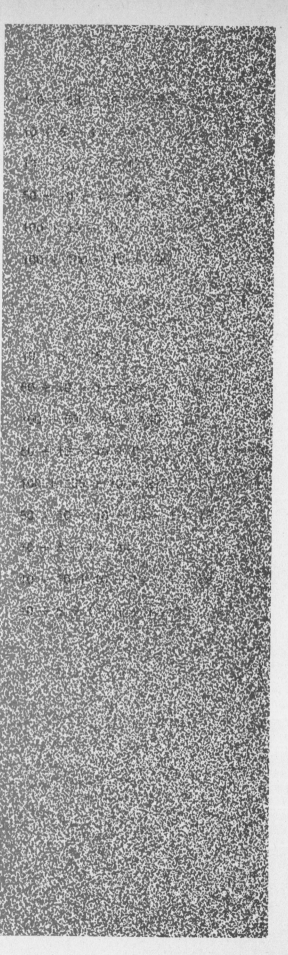

Consider the following example:

$$294$$
$$294 = 200 + 90 + 4$$
$$294 = ccxciv$$

In each of the following examples, wherever possible first break the number into its various units, and then change to Roman numerals.

1. 55

2. 101

3. 254

4. 133

5. 29

6. 14

7. 54

8. 188

9. 57

10. 90

11. 110

12. 183

13. 59

14. 203

15. 8

16. 154

17. 85

18. 175

19. 218

20. 38

21. 16

22. 75

23. 255

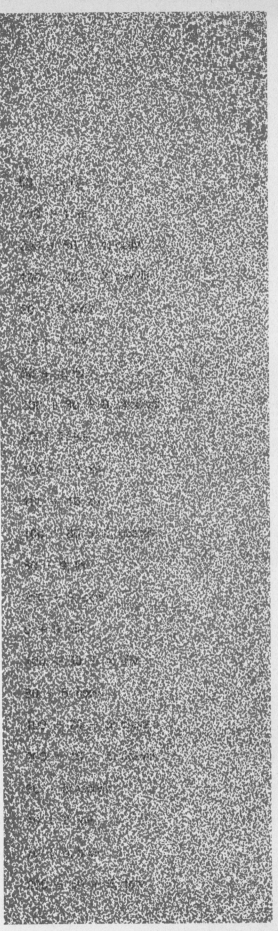

24. 21

25. 220

26. 80

27. 26

28. 224

29. 82

30. 139

Passing score is no more than *4* errors.

Appendix II

The Apothecaries' System

Section 1   Units of Weight

Even though the apothecaries' system of measurement now is rarely used by doctors in ordering medications, some drugs are still available in apothecary units. For this reason, the pharmacist and the nurse should be able to use this system and know its units. Let us first talk about the units of weight.

In the apothecaries' system, one *grain* is the weight of one drop of water, and one *dram* is the weight of a teaspoonful of water. The next unit is an *ounce,* and the largest unit is a *pound.*

Look at the following:

gr vi

"gr" is the abbreviation for grain. Whenever an abbreviation is used, the amount appears in Roman numerals following the abbreviation.

Look at the following:

6 grains

If the unit is not abbreviated, the amount is written in ordinary Arabic numbers, before the unit.

Look at the following:

$$gr\,\frac{1}{4}$$

Notice that fractions are written as fractions and appear *after* an abbreviation.

Look at the following:

gr ss

"ss" represents $\frac{1}{2}$. Therefore, gr ss means one-half of a grain.

Answer the following questions:

1. What is the weight of a drop of water?

2. What is the weight of a teaspoonful of water?

Look at the following:

$$\text{З vi}$$

"З" is the printed abbreviation for *dram*.

Notice that following an abbreviation, the amount is written in Roman numerals.

Look at the following:

$$\text{Ʒ vi or oz vi}$$

"Ʒ" or "oz" is the abbreviation for *ounce*.

Let's practice reading weights under the apothecaries' system.

What does each of the following abbreviations mean?

1. gr ii

2. З $\frac{1}{4}$

3. З iv

4. Ʒ ss

5. З iss

6. gr x

7. oz xx

8. gr xix

9. З viii

10. Ʒ xi

Notice how the abbreviation for grain is written:

$$\text{gr}$$

11. Now write the abbreviation for grain three times.

Notice how the abbreviation for dram is written:

$$\mathfrak{Z}$$

12. Now write the abbreviation for dram three times.

Notice the two ways the abbreviation for ounce is written:

$$\mathfrak{Z} \text{ or oz}$$

13. Write both abbreviations for ounce three times.

Write the abbreviations for each of the following:

14. 5 grains

15. 2 drams

16. 30 grains

17. $\frac{1}{2}$ ounce

18. $6\frac{1}{2}$ grains

19. 8 drams

20. 3 ounces

21. 7 grains

22. 24 drams

23. 19 ounces

24. $18\frac{1}{2}$ grains

25. $2\frac{1}{2}$ drams

26. 6 drams

27. 14 ounces

28. 22 grains

29. 22 ounces

30. 15 drams

Passing score is no more than *6* errors.

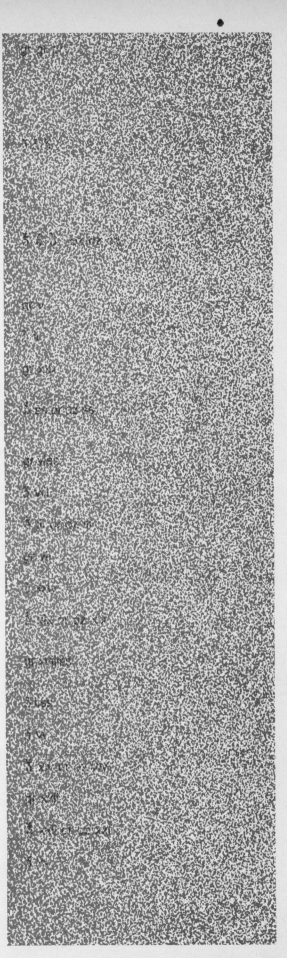

Section 2   Units of Volume

In the apothecaries' system one *minim* is the *volume* of one drop of water; one *fluidram* (fluid dram) is the *volume* of one teaspoonful of water; the next unit is a *fluidounce* (fluid ounce).

Look at the following:

m vi

"m" is the printed abbreviation for *minim*.

Look at the following:

f ℨ vii

"f ℨ" is the printed abbreviation for *fluidram*.

Look at the following:

f ℥ vi

"f ℥" is the printed abbreviation for *fluidounce*.

Let's practice reading volumes under the apothecaries' system.

What does each of the following abbreviations mean?

1. f ℨ c

2. f ℥ xviss

3. m viiss

4. f ℨ iss

5. f ℥ xxxii

6. f ℨ iiss

7. f ℥ viii

8. m xix

9. f ℨ vss

10. m xv

11. oz xxii

12. m cx

13. f ℨ ss

14. f ℥ xxss

15. f ℥ ixss

Notice how the abbreviation for minim* is written:

m

16. Write the abbreviation for minim three times.

The abbreviation for fluidram may be written in two ways:

f ℨ or ℨ

17. Write both abbreviations for fluidrams three times.

Notice how the abbreviation for fluidounce is written:

f ℥ or ℥

18. Write each abbreviation for fluidounce three times.

Write the abbreviations for each of the following:

19. 15 minims

20. $3\frac{1}{2}$ fluidrams

21. 6 fluidounces

22. 30 minims

23. $2\frac{1}{2}$ minims

24. $\frac{3}{4}$ fluidounce

25. 32 fluidrams

26. 20 fluidounces

* Note that "m" is the abbreviation for meter in the metric system and also for minim in the apothecaries' system. However, we should be able to tell which is which by its use—length in the metric system, volume in the apothecaries' system. In addition, in metric units the numbers are always Arabic and are written in front of the abbreviation; in apothecaries' units the numbers are always written after the abbreviation and are given either in Roman numerals or in fractions.

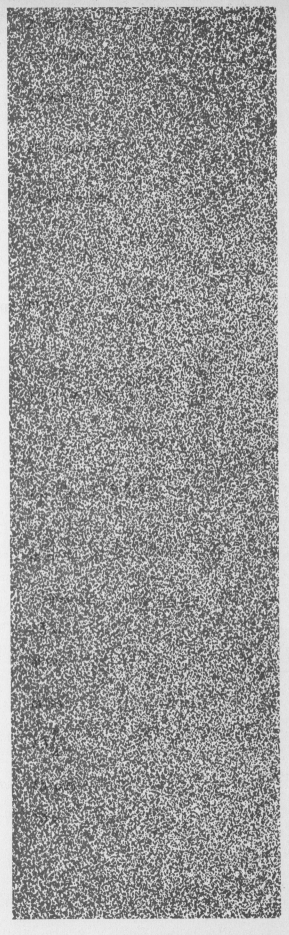

27. $\frac{1}{8}$ fluidounce

28. $1\frac{1}{2}$ fluidrams

29. 19 minims

30. $18\frac{1}{2}$ fluidrams

31. 2 fluidounces

32. $\frac{1}{4}$ fluidram

Passing score is no more than *6* errors.

Section 3 Converting Drams to Grains, and Grains to Drams

1. What is one grain?

2. What is one dram?

Consider the following question:

How many grains are in 2 drams?

The conversion unit to use is:

1 dram = 60 grains

3. If 1 dram equals 60 grains, how many grains are in 2 drams?

Whenever you want to change drams to grains, multiply the number of drams by 60.

Consider the following problem:

How many drams are in 180 grains?

4. If one dram equals 60 grains, how many drams are in 180 grains?

Whenever you want to change grains to drams, divide the number of grains by 60.

Let us try several problems.

5. Change 4 drams to grains.

6. Change 360 grains to drams.

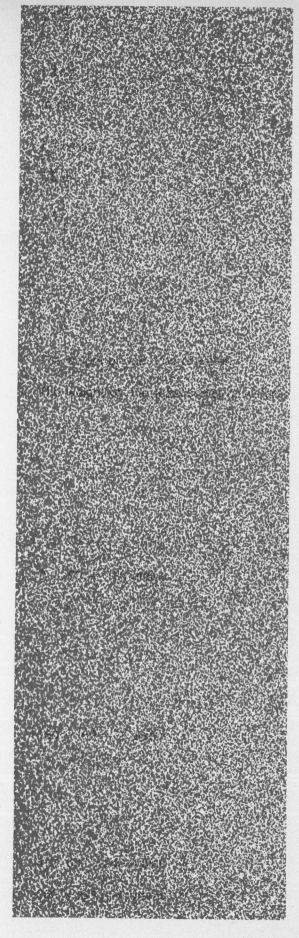

7. Change 12 drams to grains.

8. Change 480 grains to drams.

9. Change 11 drams to grains.

10. Change 1,200 grains to drams.

11. Change ʒ iii to gr.

12. Change gr xxx to ʒ.

13. Change ʒ ss to gr.

14. Change gr lx to ʒ.

15. Change ʒ ivss to gr.

Passing score is no more than *2* errors.

Section 4   Converting Ounces to Drams, and Drams to Ounces

1. What is one dram?

Consider the following question:

> *How many drams are in 3 ounces?*

The conversion unit to use is:

> **1 ounce = 8 drams**

2. If 1 ounce equals 8 drams, how many drams are in 3 ounces?

Whenever you want to change ounces to drams, multiply the number of ounces by 8.

Consider the following question:

> *How many ounces are in 24 drams?*

3. If 8 drams equal 1 ounce, how many ounces are 24 drams?

Whenever you want to change drams to ounces, divide the number of drams by 8.

Now let's try several problems.

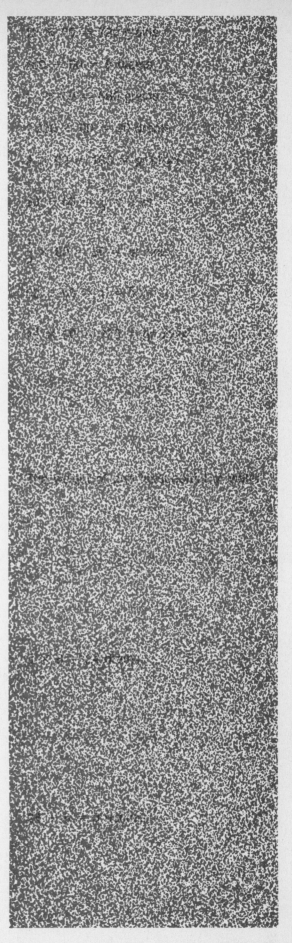

4. Change 6 ounces to drams.

5. Change 32 drams to ounces.

6. Change 5 ounces to drams.

7. Change 16 drams to ounces.

8. Change ℥ x to ℨ.

9. Change ℨ iv to ℥.

10. Change ℥ ivss to ℨ.

11. Change ℥ vii to ℨ.

12. Change ℨ vi to ℥.

13. Change ℥ xi to ℨ.

14. Change ℨ xvi to ℥.

15. Change ℥ xx to ℨ.

16. Change ℨ xii to ℥.

Passing score is no more than *3* errors.

Section 5   Review

1. How many grains is one dram?

2. How many drams is one ounce?

The conversion units needed for this review are:

> 60 grains = 1 dram
> 8 drams = 1 ounce

Let's try several problems.

1. Change ℨ lvi to ℥.

2. Change ℨ iii to gr.

3. Change gr xxx to ℨ.

4. Change gr cxx to ʒ.

5. Change ʒ ivss to gr.

6. Change ʒ iv to gr.

7. Change ℥ vi to ʒ.

8. Change ʒ xvi to ℥.

9. Change ℥ ivss to ʒ.

10. Change ʒ lxxx to ℥.

11. Change ℥ xi to ʒ.

12. Change ʒ clx to ℥.

13. Change ℥ ss to ʒ.

14. Change gr ccxl to ʒ.

15. Change ʒ lxiv to ℥.

Passing score is no more than *3* errors.

Section 6   Converting Fluidrams to Minims, and Minims to Fluidrams

1. What is a minim?

2. What is a fluidram?

Consider the following question:

How many minims are in four fluidrams?

The conversion unit to use is:

1 fluidram = 60 minims

3. If 1 fluidram equals 60 minims, how many minims are in 4 fluidrams?

Whenever you want to change fluidrams to minims, multiply the number of fluidrams by 60.

Consider the following question:

How many fluidrams are in 1,020 minims?

4. If 1 fluidram equals 60 minims, how many fluidrams are in 1,020 minims?

Whenever you want to change minims to fluidrams, divide the number of minims by 60.

Let us try several problems.

5. Change 6 fluidrams to minims.

6. Change 30 minims to fluidrams.

7. Change 10 fluidrams to minims.

8. Change 150 minims to fluidrams.

9. Change 4 fluidrams to minims.

10. Change 90 minims to fluidrams.

11. Change f $\mathfrak{Z}$ iss to m.

12. Change m lx to f $\mathfrak{Z}$.

13. Change f $\mathfrak{Z}$ v to m.

14. Change m cclxx to f $\mathfrak{Z}$.

15. Change f $\mathfrak{Z}$ ss to m.

Passing score is no more than *2* errors.

Section 7 Changing Fluidounces to Fluidrams, and Fluidrams to Fluidounces

1. What is a fluidram?

Consider the following question:

How many fluidrams are in 12 fluidounces?

The conversion unit to use is:

1 fluidounce = 8 fluidrams

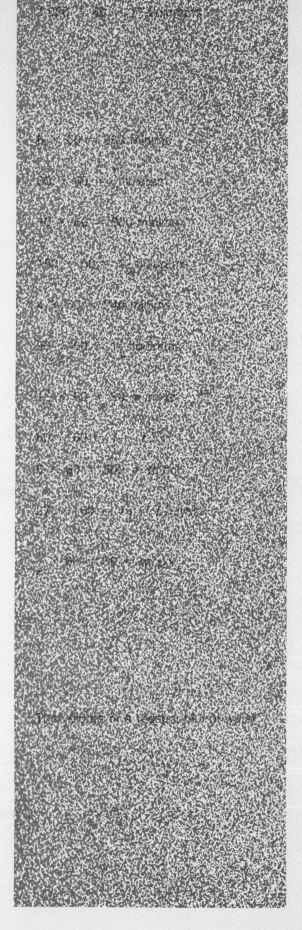

2. If 1 fluidounce equals 8 fluidrams, how many fluidrams are in 12 fluidounces?

Whenever you want to change fluidounces to fluidrams, multiply the number of fluidounces by 8.

Consider the following question:

How many fluidounces are in 24 fluidrams?

3. If 1 fluidounce equals 8 fluidrams, how many fluidounces are in 24 fluidrams?

Whenever you want to change fluidrams to fluidounces, divide the number of fluidrams by 8.

Let's try several problems.

4. Change 64 fluidrams to fluidounces.

5. Change *f* ℥ iii to *f* ʒ.

6. Change *f* ʒ lxxx to *f* ℥.

7. Change *f* ℥ ix to *f* ʒ.

8. Change *f* ʒ xvi to *f* ℥.

9. Change *f* ℥ iv to *f* ʒ.

10. Change 7$\frac{1}{2}$ fluidounces to fluidrams.

11. Change 40 fluidrams to fluidounces.

12. Change 6 fluidounces to fluidrams.

13. Change 8 fluidrams to fluidounces.

14. Change 15 fluidounces to fluidrams.

15. Change 10 fluidounces to fluidrams.

Passing score is no more than *2* errors.

Section 8   Review

1. How many minims is 1 fluidram?

2. How many fluidrams is 1 fluidounce?

3. What is the weight of one drop of water?

4. What is the volume of one drop of water?

5. What is the volume of 1 teaspoonful of water?

Note the following conversion table:

> **1 fluidram** = 60 minims
> **1 fluidounce** = 8 fluidrams

Now let's try several problems.

1. Change *f* ℥ vi to m.

2. Change m xxx to *f* ℥.

3. Change m ccclx to *f* ℥.

4. Change *f* ℥ iiss to m.

5. Change *f* ℥ v to m.

6. Change m cxx to *f* ℥.

7. Change *f* ℥ xxxii to *f* ℥.

8. Change *f* ℥ vi to *f* ℥.

9. Change *f* ℥ lxxx to *f* ℥.

10. Change *f* ℥ xx to *f* ℥.

11. Change *f* ℥ cccxx to *f* ℥.

12. Change *f* ℥ xii to *f* ℥.

13. Change *f* ℥ ii to m.

14. Change m clxxx to *f* ℥.

15. Change *f* ℥ 3¾ to m.

16. Change m xx to *f* ℥.

17. Change *f* ℥ iv to *f* ℥.

18. Change *f* ℥ xl to *f* ℥.

19. Change *f* ℥ x to *f* ℥.

20. Change *f* ℥ lxxii to *f* ℥.

Passing score is no more than *4* errors.

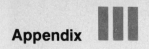

Comparison of the Apothecaries' System with the Metric System

Section 1 Apothecary and Metric Systems (Weight)

The weight conversions (approximations) are:

Metric System		Apothecaries' System
1 g	=	15 grains
4 g	=	1 dram
30 g	=	1 ounce
60 mg	=	1 grain*

You may refer to the above conversion table to answer the following questions:

1. What is the definition of 1 grain?

2. How many grains are in 1 g?

3. How many grains are in 2 g?

Whenever you want to change grams to grains, multiply the number of grams by 15.

4. How many grams equal 45 grains?

Whenever you want to change grains to grams, divide the number of grains by 15.

5. Change 5 g to grains.

6. Change gr xxx to g.†

7. Change 6 g to gr.

* See inside back cover.
† *Note:* Roman numerals are written *after* apothecary abbreviations, whereas Arabic numbers appear *before* metric abbreviations. Recall also that grams are abbreviated as g and grains as gr.

309

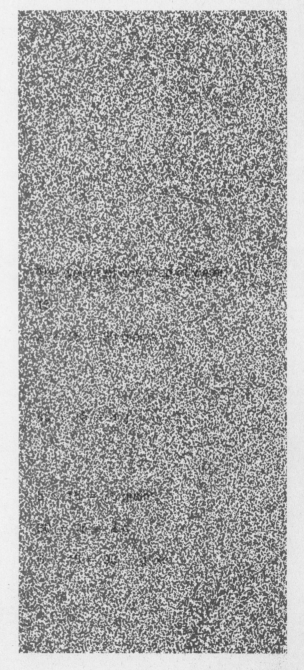

8. Change gr lx to g.

9. Change 10 g to gr.

10. Change gr x to g.

11. What is the definition of a dram?

12. How many grams equal 1 dram?

13. How many drams are in 8 grams?

Whenever you want to convert grams to drams, divide the number of drams by 4.

14. How many grams are in 2 drams?

Whenever you want to convert drams to grams, multiply the number of drams by 4.

15. Change $3\frac{1}{4}$ to g.

16. Change 40 g to ℥.

17. Change ℥ xiv to g.

18. Change 12 g to ℥.

19. Change ℥ xi to g.

20. Change 88 g to ℥.

21. Change ℥ ii to g.

22. Change 68 g to ℥.

23. Change ℥ xx to g.

24. Change 2 g to ℥.

25. Change ℥ ix to g.

26. How many grams are in 1 ounce?

27. How many grams are in 2 ounces?

Whenever you want to change ounces to grams, multiply the number of ounces by 30.

28. How many ounces are in 90 grams?

Whenever you want to change grams to ounces, divide the number of grams by 30.

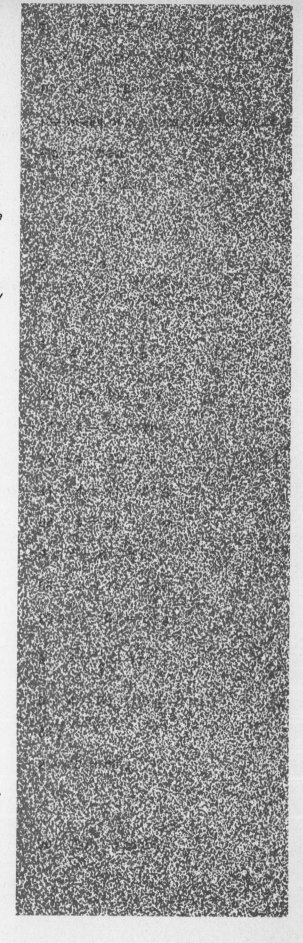

29. Change 90 g to ℥.

30. Change ℥ ii to g.

31. Change 120 g to ℥.

32. Change ℥ viii to g.

33. Change ℥ iii to g.

34. Change 180 g to ℥.

35. Change 15 g to ℥.

36. Change ℥ x to g.

37. Change 1 g to ℥.

38. Change ℥ ix to g.

39. Change 7 g to gr.

40. Change 2 g to gr.

41. Change 60 g to ℥.

42. Change ℥ viii to g.

43. Change 270 g to ℥.

44. Change gr xlv to g.

45. Change 4 g to gr.

46. Change gr ccxxv to g.

47. Change 2.5 g to gr.

48. Change ℨ vii to g.

49. Change 18 g to ℥.

50. Change ℨ ii to g.

Passing score is no more than *7* errors.

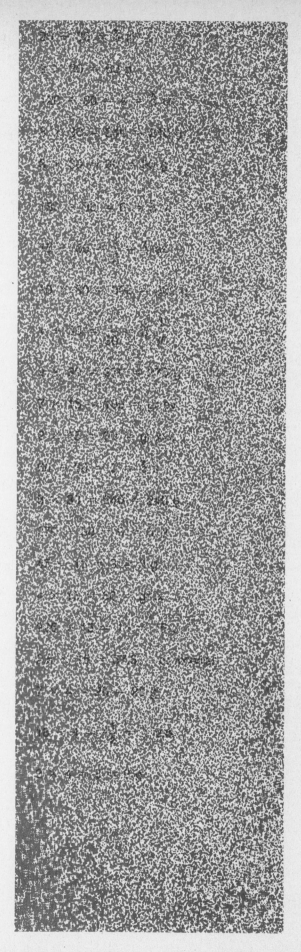

Section 2 Apothecary and Metric Systems (Volume)

The volume conversions (approximations) are:

Metric System		Apothecaries' System
1 ml (cc)	=	15 minims
4 ml (cc)	=	1 dram (fluidram)
30 ml (cc)	=	1 ounce (fluidounce)
500 ml (cc)	=	1 pint
1 liter	=	1 quart

You may refer to the above conversion table in order to answer the following questions:

1. What is the definition of 1 minim?

2. How many minims are in 1 milliliter?

3. How many minims are in 2 milliliters?

Whenever you want to change milliliters to minims, multiply the number of milliliters by 15.

4. How many milliliters are in 45 minims?

Whenever you want to change minims to milliliters, divide the number of minims by 15.

5. How many minims are in 4 cc?

Whenever you want to change cubic centimeters to minims, multiply the number of cubic centimeters by 15.

6. How many cubic centimeters are in 45 minims?

Whenever you want to change minims to cubic centimeters, divide the number of minims by 15.

7. Change 4 ml to m.

8. Change m xlv to ml.

9. Change 8 ml to m.

10. Change m ccxl to ml.

11. Change 2 cc to m.

12. Change m xc to cc.

13. Change 7 cc to m.

14. Change m ccx to ml.

15. Change $\frac{1}{2}$ cc to m.

16. What is the definition of 1 fluidram?

17. How many milliliters or cubic centimeters are in 1 fluidram?

18. How many milliliters are in 2 fluidrams?

Whenever you want to change fluidrams to milliliters, multiply the number of fluidrams by 4.

19. How many cubic centimeters are in 3 fluidrams?

Whenever you want to change fluidrams to cubic centimeters, multiply the number of fluidrams by 4.

20. How many fluidrams are in 8 cc?

Whenever you want to change cubic centimeters to fluidrams, divide the number of cubic centimeters by 4.

21. How many fluidrams are in 12 ml?

Whenever you want to change milliliters to fluidrams, divide the number of milliliters by 4.

22. Change f ℨ iii to cc.

23. Change 16 cc to f ℨ.

24. Change f ℨ x to cc.

25. Change ℥ ii to g.

26. Change 180 g to ℥.

27. Change ℥ xi to g.

28. Change 24 cc to f ℨ.

29. Change f ℨ xvi to cc.

30. Change 10 cc to f ℨ.

31. Change f ℨ iv to cc.

32. Change 48 cc to f ℨ.

33. Change 2.5 g to gr.

34. Change 120 g to ℥.

35. Change f ℨ vii to cc.

36. Change $f \, ʒ$ iii to ml.

37. Change 16 ml to $f \, ʒ$.

38. Change $f \, ʒ$ x to ml.

39. Change 24 ml to $f \, ʒ$.

40. Change 10 ml to $f \, ʒ$.

41. Change $f ʒ$ iv to ml.

42. Change 48 ml to $f \, ʒ$.

43. Change $f \, ʒ$ xvi to cc.

44. Change gr xxx to g.

45. Change 3 g to gr.

46. Change gr lxxv to g.

47. Change 4 g to gr.

48. Change gr ccc to g.

49. How many milliliters or cubic centimeters are in 1 fluid-ounce?

50. How many milliliters or cubic centimeters are in 2 fluid-ounces?

Whenever you want to change fluidounces to cubic centimeters or milliliters, multiply the number of fluidounces by 30.

51. How many fluidounces are in 90 cc or 90 ml?

Whenever you want to change cubic centimeters or milliliters to fluidounces, divide the number of cc or ml by 30.

52. Change $f \, ℥$ c to cc.

53. Change $f \, ℥$ c to ml.

54. Change 60 cc to $f \, ℥$.

55. Change $f \, ℥$ v to cc.

56. Change $f \, ℥$ viiss to ml.

57. Change 15 ml to $f \, ℥$.

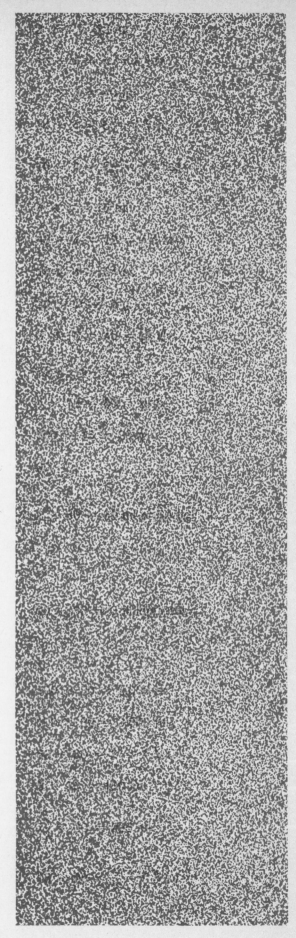

58. Change $f\,\mathfrak{Z}$ iv to cc.

59. Change $f\,\mathfrak{Z}\,\dfrac{2}{3}$ to cc.

60. Change $f\,\mathfrak{Z}$ iii to ml.

61. Change 240 cc to $f\,\mathfrak{Z}$.

62. Change $f\,\mathfrak{Z}$ vi to cc.

63. Change 25 ml to $f\,\mathfrak{Z}$.

64. Change 150 ml to $f\,\mathfrak{Z}$.

65. Change $f\,\mathfrak{Z}$ xii to cc.

Passing score is no more than *7* errors.

Section 3 Metric-Apothecary Conversions Using Milligram Weight

Consider the following question:

How many milligrams equal one-half grain?

The conversion unit to use is:

1 grain = 60 milligrams*

1. If 1 grain equals 60 milligrams, how many milligrams does $\dfrac{1}{2}$ grain equal?

To change grains to milligrams, multiply the number of grains by 60.

2. How many grains are in 120 milligrams?

To change milligrams to grains, divide the number of milli-grams by 60.

3. Change gr vi to mg.

4. Change 120 mg to gr.

5. Change gr x to mg.

6. Change 300 mg to gr.

* See inside back cover.

7. Change gr iv to mg.

8. Change 0.2 mg to gr.

9. Change gr ii to mg.

10. Change 0.06 mg to gr.

11. Change gr $\frac{1}{5}$ to mg.

12. Change gr $\frac{1}{100}$ to mg.

13. Change gr $\frac{1}{600}$ to mg.

Passing score is no more than *1* error.

Section 4   Medications from Tablets

Consider the following problem:

Give $\frac{1}{2}$ grain of phenobarbital from phenobarbital tablets 30 mg.

1. Write the equation for determining the number of tablets to give the patient.

2. Substitute the known values.

3. However, you cannot divide grains by milligrams. Therefore, either change grains to milligrams, or change milligrams to grains, and solve for the number of tablets. While the answer should be the same for either method, the preferred change should be to the metric unit.

Solve each of the following problems for the correct number of tablets.

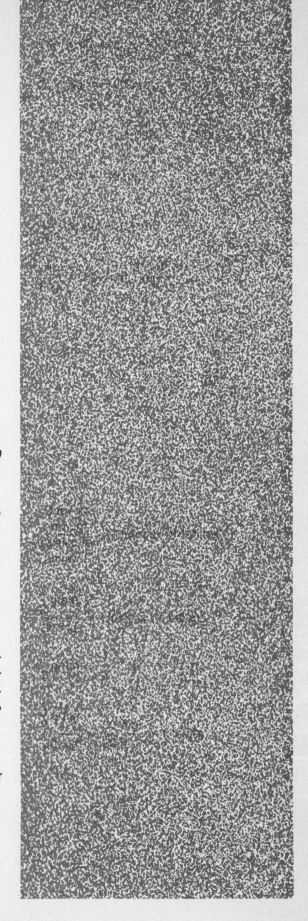

4. Give 5 mg of a drug from tablets gr $\frac{1}{12}$.

5. Give gr $\frac{1}{150}$ from tablets gr $\frac{1}{100}$.

6. Give gr $\frac{1}{100}$ from tablets 0.6 mg.

Passing score is no more than *1* error.

Section 5   Review

1. Change 15 g to gr.

2. Change ℥ ix to g.

3. Change 150 g to ℥.

4. Change 120 mg to gr.

5. Change 0.5 ml to minims.

6. Change 48 ml to f ℥.

7. Change 15 cc to f ℥.

8. Change gr xxx to g.

9. Change 12 g to ℥.

10. Change ℥ xi to g.

11. Change gr lx to g.

12. Change m cxx to ml.

13. Change f ʒ x to ml.

14. Change f ℥ x to ml.

15. Change 0.6 mg to gr.

16. Change gr $\dfrac{1}{150}$ to mg.

17. Change 4 g to gr.

18. Change 88 g to ʒ.

19. Change 300 g to ℥.

20. Change 90 mg to gr.

21. Change 2 ml to m.

22. Change 80 cc to f ʒ.

23. Change 120 cc to f ℥.

24. Change 0.1 mg to gr.

25. Change gr $\dfrac{1}{1,000}$ to mg.

Passing score is no more than *4* errors.

Apothecaries' System Practice Test No. 1

1. Change gr cxx to ʒ.

2. Change 120 mg to gr.

3. Change f ʒ iss to m.

4. Change 60 g to ℥.

5. Change gr clxxx to g.

6. Change ʒ ss to gr.

7. Change ℥ iss to g.

8. Change ℈ iii to ʒ.

9. Change 2 ml to m.

10. Change 2 ml to f ʒ.

11. Change f ℥ ii to f ʒ.

12. Change ℥ ss to g.

13. Change m xc to f ʒ.

14. Change 3 g to ℈.

15. Change 2 g to gr.

16. Change ℈ $\frac{1}{4}$ to gr.

17. Change gr ss to mg.

18. Change m xlv to ml.

19. Change f ℈ ss to f ℥.

20. Change 20 ml to f ℥.

21. Change f ℈ $\frac{1}{4}$ to ml.

22. Change f ℥ ii to ml.

23. To give gr $\frac{1}{100}$ from tablets 0.6 mg, give _____ .

24. To give gr $\frac{1}{600}$ from tablets 0.05 mg, give _____ .

25. To give gr v from tablets 300 mg, give _____ .

Apothecaries' System Practice Test No. 2

1. Change 180 mg to gr.

2. Change 90 g to ℥.

3. Change gr ccxl to ℈.

4. Change ℈ ss to ℥.

5. Change gr xlv to g.

6. Change f ℥ iiss to m.

7. Change 6 ml to m.

8. Change ℈ ii to gr.

9. Change 0.5 g to gr.

10. Change ℈ ss to g.

11. Change gr iv to mg.

12. Change 2.5 ml to m.

13. Change m xxx to f ℈.

14. Change f ℈ iii to f ℥.

15. Change f ℥ iii to f ℈.

16. Change ℈ iii to gr.

17. Change 8 g to ℈.

18. Change ℥ ii to g.

19. Change m xxx to ml.

20. Change f ℈ iss to ml.

21. Change f ℥ iss to ml.

22. Change 10 ml to f ℥.

23. To give gr $\frac{1}{100}$ from tablets 0.3 mg, give _____ .

24. To give gr x from tablets 300 mg, give _____ .

25. To give gr $\frac{1}{600}$ from tablets 0.1 mg, give _____ .

Apothecaries' System Practice Test No. 3

1. Change f ℈ ss to m.

2. Change gr x to ℈.

3. Change 45 g to ℥.

4. Change 2 mg to gr.

5. Change ʒ xvi to ℥.

6. Change gr xxx to g.

7. Change ʒ v to gr.

8. Change ʒ iv to g.

9. Change ℥ ss to g.

10. Change 4 ml to m.

11. Change f ℥ ii to f ʒ.

12. Change m x to f ʒ.

13. Change 8 ml to f ʒ.

14. Change ʒ iii to gr.

15. Change 10 g to ʒ.

16. Change m lx to ml.

17. Change 4 g to gr.

18. Change f ʒ ii to ml.

19. Change f ʒ ii to f ℥.

20. Change 75 ml to f ℥.

21. Change gr ii to mg.

22. Change f ℥ iv to ml.

23. To give 0.6 mg from tablets gr $\frac{1}{100}$, give _____ .

24. To give gr $\frac{1}{10}$ from tablets 12 mg, give _____ .

25. To give gr ii from tablets 120 mg, give _____ .

Apothecaries' System Practice Test No. 4

1. Change 15 ml to f ℥.

2. Change 2 mg to gr.

3. Change f ʒ $\frac{1}{4}$ to m.

4. Change 90 g to ℥.

5. Change ʒ ii to gr.

6. Change gr xv to g.

7. Change ʒ iv to g.

8. Change ʒ iv to ℥.

9. Change gr xx to ʒ.

10. Change 10 ml to m.

11. Change 10 ml to f ʒ.

12. Change f ℥ v to f ʒ.

13. Change ℥ iii to g.

14. Change m lx to f ʒ.

15. Change 12 g to ʒ.

16. Change 0.8 g to gr.

17. Change ʒ iss to gr.

18. Change gr $\frac{1}{10}$ to mg.

19. Change m xxx to ml.

20. Change f ʒ ii to f ℥.

21. Change f ʒ ii to ml.

22. Change 45 ml to f ℥.

23. To give gr $\frac{1}{20}$ from tablets 3 mg, give _____ .

24. To give gr ss from tablets 15 mg, give _____ .

25. To give gr $\frac{1}{200}$ from tablets 0.3 mg, give _____ .

Abbreviations Used in Prescriptions and Doctors' Orders

Common Abbreviation	Computer Printout Abbreviation	Latin Derivation	Meaning
a̅ a̅	AA	ana	of each
a.c.	AC	ante cibum	before meals
ad lib.	AD LIB	ad libitum	as desired
aq.	AQ	aqua	water
b.i.d.	BID	bis in die	twice a day
c̅.	C	cum	with
D/W	D/W		dextrose and water
et	&	et	and
gtt.	GTT	gutta	drop(s)
h.s.	HS	hora somni	at bedtime
IM	IM		intramuscularly
IV	IV		intravenously
IVP	IVP		IV push
IVPB	IVPB		IV piggyback
mEq	MEQ		milliequivalent
N/S	N/S		normal saline
O.D.	OD	oculus dexter	right eye
O.S.	OS	oculus sinister	left eye
p.c.	PC	post cibum	after meals
p.o.	PO	per os	by mouth
p.r.n.	PRN	pro re nata	when necessary
q.a.m.	QAM		every morning
q.d.	QD	quaque die	every day
q.h.	QH	quaque hora	every hour
q.2h.	Q2H	quaque 2 hora	every 2 hours
q.3h.	Q3H	quaque 3 hora	every 3 hours
q.i.d.	QID	quatuor in die	four times a day
q.p.m.	QPM		every evening
q.s.	QS	quatum sufficit	as much as is required
s̅.	S	sine	without
s.o.s.	SOS	si opus sit	if necessary
stat.	STAT	statim	immediately
subq	SUBQ		subcutaneously
t.i.d.	TID	ter in die	three times a day
ut dict	UD	ut dictum	as directed
W/A	W/A		when awake